Of This Sad Time

My Wife's Journey Through Breast Cancer

Karl D. Stephan

Stephan Publishing, San Marcos, Texas

ISBN-13: 978-0-9970283-2-4
ISBN-10: 0997028327

The weight of this sad time we must obey;

Speak what we feel, not what we ought to say.

King Lear, *V, III*

Contents

Foreword

This is the story of my wife's fight with breast cancer and my role in that fight. Shortly after I finished writing this book in 2004, the Iraq war began. Most Americans have never experienced war personally. But every year, breast cancer attacks more than 200,000 women in the United States alone. Fighting cancer is a lot like being drafted into a war zone. Your life is in danger, you didn't ask to be there, you'd better learn how to do certain things pretty quick or you'll die, and even some of the things designed to fight for you can kill you if you're not careful. We had to learn a lot about breast cancer in a short time. If you or someone you love has breast cancer, I hope that reading about our experience can help you with yours.

Chapter 1

Orphaned At 30

In 1971, I was seventeen. All I thought about then was circuits and electronics and cool stuff you could do with them. I hung out with a bunch of guys who liked to build machines that made six-inch sparks and melted copper wires. Our gang's official name was Explorer Post 292. My father called it the Boy Sprouts.

Every so often, we'd go on tours of power plants and factories. That winter we took a tour of the Texas Instruments plant in Dallas. The tour took all day. That night I got home about eight. When I got home, my father told me that my mother had cancer. I knew she was going in the hospital that day. I just decided to go on the tour instead of waiting around the hospital.

They cut off her breast as soon as they found out it was cancerous. She didn't know any of this until she woke up after the surgery.

My father kept a pile of Playboy magazines under their bed. My mother read them for the interviews. He looked at the pictures. This may have had something to do with my mother's decision to get large implants after her surgery. They failed. She went through several more painful surgeries.

In 1979, the cancer came back. My mother started

chemotherapy. By that time I had married and was living in Atlanta, Georgia. My mother flew out from Texas and we took her to a restaurant in an old Southern mansion. My wife took a picture of her and me on the front steps of the place. My mother is smiling a big smile. But she is stooped and shorter than me by a good six inches.

Two months later, I got a phone call at work. My father said if I wanted to see her again, to come back to Texas now. We got on a plane and went to the hospital. She was weak and had on a fake-looking wig. We talked a little bit, and then her mouth got dry and she sucked some water through a straw. We left the room.

The next day when we came in, she was delirious. Her wig was off and the bare scalp had some purple marks on it. We stayed at the hospital all day and into the evening. Around 11:30 that night she began to moan. Then she vomited some black blood. I ran out into the hall for a nurse. The nurse went into the room. A few minutes later my father came out with his hands in his pockets. "She's gone," he said. She was fifty.

Three years later, my father began to cough up blood. He had smoked all his adult life. His doctor took X-rays and found a mass near the center of his chest. He went into surgery. The surgeon found a tumor where the two main bronchia join to form the windpipe. It was inoperable. His doctor believed he could last about a year. This was in March of 1983.

The following March, we were living in Massachusetts where I had a teaching job. We made plans to visit my father during the spring break. I called him on the Saturday a week before the break. He sounded tired and said he wasn't feeling good. But he was scheduled to go in for some experimental surgery the following Tuesday. He said, "I'll either die or get better."

On Tuesday, I was in my office working at the computer. It was snowing heavily. My department head, a man named Bob, knocked on the door. I let him in. He was accompanied by a colleague of mine, a kindhearted ageless Swede who said nothing. Bob said, "Your father had an operation today and it failed. I'm sorry." No one but a doctor he didn't know that well was with him when he died. He was fifty-seven.

By the time I was thirty, I knew about as much about cancer as someone can know who hasn't lived around a cancer patient day after day and who hasn't had it himself. I found out later that that's not very much. When you watch somebody die, you don't learn much about how they lived. But I did learn not to put off going to see people I knew who had cancer. Death is one appointment you can't reschedule.

Chapter 2

Pam And the Diving Pig

My wife. Her name is Pam, which is short for Pamela. Her middle name is Louise. Sometimes her father used to call her "Pamie-Lou" and it embarrassed her. When she married me she was glad to drop the Louise and just be Pam Stephan.

The old knights used to joust anybody who insulted their lady love. Jousting was sort of like a duel, only with horses and spears instead of guns. It was serious business. No knight worthy of the name would ever say anything bad about his own lady love. So I won't either. But she's human.

She's real smart. Likes movies. Old movies in particular. That's one reason I married her. She took life a little more seriously than most of the other women her age. We knew each other for two years while we were finishing college in different states. Wrote letters back and forth. One day when I was back in Texas working at a mobile radio factory, I picked her up in my white VW Beetle. We drove over to Dallas and saw the old Disney cartoon "Fantasia." On the way back we decided to get married.

We never slept together before we got married. VW Beetles are not conducive to necking. We got pretty hot and heavy standing in her folks' hallway a few times. Eventually her dad would find some excuse to come out in the hall and make some noise. I got the message. He kept a shotgun in the back closet, and he was the kind of guy who knew how to use it.

I like looking at women's bodies as well as the next guy. I liked looking at hers. We went swimming a few times before we were married. She wore a two-piece suit that gave me a good idea of what there was. Playboy wouldn't have her, but there are other things in life besides large breasts.

Neither one of us knew what we were doing on our wedding night. She was very nice about it. When there's a will, there's a way. We kept practicing. We got better.

I used to believe in magic. Here's what I mean. I believed that once you got married, no other woman would ever look attractive to you again. The strange thing was, I didn't know I believed this until I got married. The day after our wedding night in Waco, Texas, we drove to San Marcos.

San Marcos is a small town halfway between Austin and San Antonio. There was an amusement park there called Aquarena Springs. The star attraction was Arnold the Diving Pig. We watched the pig dive into the springs. There was also a university there. We went for a walk in a public park. It was a warm day. Lots of young co-eds were walking around in miniskirts and tight tops. I still liked looking at them. Just as much as the day before.

What the hell? I thought. This isn't working. I'm not supposed to like looking at other women any more. But I sure did.

I don't believe in that kind of magic any more. Nothing is automatic about staying married. There's nothing automatic about fighting a bull, either. Both take practice. And one is just about as hard as the other, but for different reasons.

Chapter 3

A Close Call

Fast forward to early 1994. Pam had her own career by that time. She learned how to do technical drawings on a computer. A staff friend of hers, another Pam, taught her how to write pages for a new thing called the Internet. In the middle of all this her health plan told her to go get a breast exam. She never had a breast exam before. She was thirty-eight. It's time. Some people would say past time.

Nobody normal likes to go to doctors. But some people dislike it less than others. Pam really disliked it. She went anyway. Her nurse practitioner had a funny feeling about the manual exam and ordered a mammogram. The mammogram had "microcalcifications." In English, that means small pieces of rock that can mean cancer. They said to come back in six months for another exam. Fine.

We went on a trip in July. When we got back, there was a message on the answering machine that said her grandmother had died. We went back to Texas from where we're living in Massachusetts for the funeral. Her grandmother was in her eighties and died of old age. Like Pam wants to.

The day after we got back from the funeral, Pam went in for the manual exam and mammogram. More microcalcifications. They scheduled surgery, a "needle biopsy." It wasn't what I thought it

6

would be. The surgeon goes in with a needle and watches an X-ray to get it close to the suspicious area. Then he turns off the X-ray and goes in with whatever he needs to remove some tissue and sends it to the lab. Then they do whatever the lab results tell them to, later.

Before the biopsy, Pam talked to some of her few women friends. One or two had this sort of procedure and it turned out fine. We also knew a woman who had breast cancer–six years earlier. She was fine now, minus a breast.

A few days before the surgery, a woman named Ginger showed up in Pam's office. Ginger went to a church we had visited a few times. She worked in the same college Pam did, but Pam didn't know her that well. Ginger put her hands on Pam and prayed against the devil and all his works, that the Holy Spirit would fill Pam and all spirits of infirmity, sickness, and cancer would depart, in Jesus' name, Amen. Pam didn't quite know what to say to this.

The next day I drove Pam to the hospital. We were late because of some foulup with the HMO and I drove a little too fast. She was nervous. We registered at the desk and sat down in the waiting room. They called Pam's name. I squeezed her arm and let her go. Then I tried to sit there and read *King Lear*.

The early part of the play is about Lear and his three daughters. Lear wants to retire but not let go of all his power. He's asked each of his daughters how much they love him. Goneril and Regan gush extravagant flattery. But all Cordelia says is that she loves him as much as is his due. He throws a fit and tells her he was going to give her a third of his kingdom, but not now. The Duke of Burgundy has been hanging around, nosing out the prospects for a good match. He had his eye on Cordelia, but when he finds out she's going to get cut off without a cent, Burgundy says to her, "I am sorry, then you have so lost a father / That you must lose a husband."

Cordelia gives as good as she gets: "Peace be with Burgundy! / Since that respects of fortune are his love, I shall not be his wife."

I wondered if having one breast instead of two falls under the category of "respects of fortune."

I heard the door open, much too soon. It was Pam. She was

7

smiling.

"What happened?" I asked.

"It's done. Let's go home. They didn't operate. Ginger's prayer has been answered."

The earlier mammograms were done on a less fancy machine than the hospital had. When the hospital's radiologist looked for what the earlier films showed, he couldn't find anything. It just looked like "adenosis," whatever that is. They tell us it's not cancer. So they said just to go home and they would look again in six months and then if nothing bad showed up, they would go back to once a year exams. We were relieved. For the next six years, they looked every year and never found anything worth operating on. In the meantime, Pam tells whoever will listen how Ginger's prayer saved her from cancer surgery.

Chapter 4

Suspense In Texas

My sister still lived in Texas. It is hard to persuade Texans to fly to Massachusetts for Christmas. So we flew to Texas every winter for Christmas. And every year, when we flew back and got off the plane in Connecticut and walked outside into the cold and ice and sleet falling down our necks, we'd turn to each other and say, "Why'd we come back?"

Finally I decided to do something about it. I began to look for jobs in Texas. My trouble is I'm too specialized. If I were a nurse or an auto mechanic it would be no big deal. But college-level teaching jobs in electrical engineering don't show up every day. In 1998, Baylor had an opening. I interviewed there. They seemed to like me. Then they asked me if I was a Baptist. I couldn't say I was. They have a little rule that says at least half of their professors have to be Baptist. So for every non-Baptist professor they hire, they have to find a Baptist. I wasn't going to help them there. They finally found a Baptist and hired him instead.

A year later, I found out about a fellowship program the National Science Foundation runs. It paid for a year at another university. I called up a professor at the University of Texas at Austin and asked his help to get the fellowship. We wrote a proposal and got the money. So that meant Pam and I could move to Austin for a year. Since we didn't know whether we were coming back, we took half our stuff with us and locked the other half in the basement. That way, no matter what happened we'd only have to move the other half.

The fellowship time was great. We moved to Austin in the summer of 1999. There was only one little hitch. We had to buy our own health insurance. I hunted around and found a place that sold insurance at a yearly rate we could afford. As soon as you used it once, they canceled the policy right afterward. They told you this right up front. But as long as you didn't use it, you could say you had health insurance. Their office was in a building in downtown Austin. On the way out of the building, I opened the door onto the sidewalk. A big young woman on a bicycle came tearing down the sidewalk and nearly knocked me over. If I had showed up two seconds earlier, I would have blown our health insurance for the year.

We didn't have a regular family doctor that year. That was fine with Pam. We liked being back in Texas so much that around the first of the year 2000 we decided to stay, one way or another. She started looking for a job. Two months later she found one at the University of Texas. Their College of Communication wanted a webmaster. She was just what they needed. She started work on the day after Valentine's Day.

Now she had health insurance. But she didn't bother to find a doctor. What she found was a nurse practitioner. I never met the woman. She was into herbs and whatnot. And she was cheap. Pam had had some pains here and there. The woman recommended some herbal medication that seemed to do some good.

In May of 2000, I saw an ad for a teaching job at Southwest Texas State University in San Marcos. By then, the diving pig had retired and the amusement park had gone bust. But the university was still there and looking for someone like me. I called them up. We had lunch. They seemed like a good bunch of guys. In June I left for a six-week seminar in Michigan. Later in the month they called me to interview with them on the first week of July. I flew back, had the interview, stayed over the Fourth of July weekend, and flew back up to Michigan to finish the seminar. A couple of weeks later, they called me to offer me the job.

I accepted. We were staying in Texas.

Now both of us had regular jobs. I encouraged Pam to find a regular doctor. She wasn't interested and seemed happy with the nurse practitioner. In the same office, there was a doctor who signed prescriptions. He was also rumored to be married to the nurse practitioner.

A year went by. Pam enjoyed her job. She met a lot of creative people she liked. In her spare time, she and her new friends produced a one-minute video to answer the question "What is art?" for a local public TV station that ran a contest for the best videos. Her video was one of a dozen to win a public screening. That was in August 2001.

On a Tuesday in September, I was sitting at my computer in my office. The phone rang. It was Pam. She said the government was being attacked and should she come home or should I come up there? I thought she was joking. But then she said she was serious. Planes were crashing into the World Trade Center towers and the Pentagon.

I went out to see what was going on. They had a small TV running in the main office. There were the towers, blazing away. Nobody got much else done that day.

The month after that, Pam went to see her nurse practitioner about some breast pain she'd been having. The lady did a manual exam and said it was nothing serious, probably hormonal. She gave her some advice about herbal remedies, and that was that.

It didn't go away. There was a lump of notable size in her left breast. It was beginning to pull in the nipple some. This had happened with my mother. I knew the sensible thing to do was for her to have a mammogram. I asked her to do it. She said her nurse practitioner didn't think it was needed. I said it wouldn't cost that much. I got down on my knees and begged her. She told me to quit being silly.

After some looking around, we had settled on a small Episcopal church in Austin to attend. Pam had just been asked to be on the vestry committee, which is the closest thing an Episcopal church has to a board of directors. On the first Sunday in March of 2002, before Pam knew she had a problem, we heard that Geneva Hutson was ill and in the hospital. Pam knew Geneva was the vestry committee secretary. She was a small, bright-eyed woman who seemed to be either in charge of everything or to know who was. It was unusual for her to be ill, so we decided to go up and see her after church.

We met our pastor Father Len and his wife Nancy in the elevator of the hospital. They said Geneva had some kind of stomach problem. When we got to her room, her husband Walter was there. He was a big, shambling man with old-fashioned rimless glasses. When we arrived, Geneva told us that they were worried about a tumor on her liver. She had had some strange fevers and other symptoms. She seemed to be in a good state of mind. Father Len gave her the Eucharist, we chatted for a while until her son came in, and then we went home. Later in the week we got a call from someone who told us that Geneva had stomach cancer which had spread to her liver.

The following Wednesday, Pam called to set up an appointment to have a mammogram. She put it off until after our trip to the Gulf on spring break, which came later in March.

Our vacation to the Gulf was a strange trip. We bought tickets on a double-decker passenger boat that went out near the whooping-crane nesting grounds off Corpus Christi Bay. The morning was foggy and cool for March. The fog cleared as we went out in the Gulf. It came back as we moved into an inlet and followed a channel toward the nests.

Whooping cranes mate for life. The female usually lays two eggs every year. When this happens, the parents feed one chick and leave the other one to die. The whooping cranes nearly died out in the 1940s. Then Franklin Roosevelt established a sanctuary for them along the Gulf near Rockport. There were only about 40 of them then. Now there are over 300.

As we approached the grassy shoreline, the pilot cut the boat's motor. It drifted slowly toward land. I pointed our binoculars toward the shore. I saw two tall white birds hunting for food in the shallows. These were the whooping cranes. The fog made it hard to see them against the whitish background. About fifty feet was as close as we got. We took pictures with a telephoto lens. You can see two tall white birds in one or two of the photos. They don't look as tall in the pictures as they do in real life. We drove back to San Marcos after a couple of days in Rockport. It was still foggy and cool.

Chapter 5

The Mammogram

Pam went to have her mammogram the following Wednesday, March 20. I couldn't be with her because I had to teach a lab in San Marcos. She went to a radiologist in Austin.

Around noon I got back to my office. There was a message on my phone. It was Pam. She was at home. She sounded upset. I got in my car and drove home.

What they usually do at a radiologist is to get you in position, take their pictures, and then keep you there until they see if they got what they wanted. Then they send you away and you find out the results later. That was what had always happened before.

This time was different. A woman technician got Pam in the room, squeezed the members in question, and took some pictures. Then she had Pam lie down, applied an ultrasound probe, and took more pictures. She went away. There were signs in the room saying not to ask anyone about the results, that they'd be sent to your doctor, so Pam put on her clothes and got ready to leave.

Then the door opened. A man came into the room. He said he was the radiologist. He thought she might have breast cancer. He was worried about an ill-defined mass in the left breast. He told her to see her family doctor right away about setting up a biopsy. Only she didn't have a family doctor. Just the nurse practitioner. Pam was not in any mood to go back to her.

She stayed on the access roads most of the way back from Austin to San Marcos. She was too upset to trust herself to drive on the interstate.

After she told me all this, she cried. I cried with her. It was bad.

A few days later she offered to let me feel it. Feeling your wife's breast for cancer is completely different than feeling it for other reasons. It was easy to tell there was a hard ball a little less than an inch across, with sort of spiny projections on it. There it was, right between her and me. If we didn't do something about it, it would kill her.

She told a few people: an old friend in Massachusetts, a new friend at our church in Austin, and some friends who live in North Carolina. She called the nurse practitioner back just long enough to get a recommendation for a surgeon. She recommended a Dr. Harvey Worchel, whom we would meet the following week.

I wasn't as surprised as Pam was. But it wasn't my breast.

I had a lot of thoughts around that time. I thought of how my mother died. I thought of what my life would be like if Pam died soon. Even if you decide not to think about something, you think about it when you remember not to think about it. I went through a long process of consciously catching myself thinking such thoughts and telling myself not to think them. Gradually, after a lot of practice, the thoughts didn't come back so often.

They would still come back from time to time when I was tired or discouraged. Nowadays, I hardly ever have trouble with thoughts like that. It is easier to believe that Pam will be around for a while. Back then, after her first diagnosis, we knew only the word "cancer." And for all we knew, she might die soon.

My nephew Matt was going to be baptized on the Sunday after Pam's mammogram. On the drive up to Fort Worth, we decided not to burden the occasion with our bad news. In the Disciples of Christ church, baptism takes place at the age of understanding, which most people take to be about twelve.

My sister attends the same church where my mother and father attended. It is a large, well-organized church of middle and upper class people. When the time came, Matt waded into the water of the baptistry and got dunked. Baptism is a symbol of death and resurrection. You put your trust in the preacher as a representative of Christ. He grabs you and plunges you underwater. If he decides to keep you there, and you weigh eighty pounds and he weighs 160, there's not much you can do about it. But he always pulls you up again.

I called my sister once we got back to San Marcos to let her know we were okay. She said Pam seemed subdued.

Chapter 6

The Biopsy

Dr. Harvey Worchel is from Missouri. He would look natural dressed in denim overalls and a straw hat, chewing on a piece of hay while he explained exactly what went wrong with your $130,000 harvester and how he was going to fix it. He talks the same way about what goes wrong in your body and how to fix it.

I went with Pam this time. (Eventually I made it a rule that I would go with her to any appointment at which she might receive bad news. That rule caused me to go with her to many appointments in the next few months.) Dr. Worchel explained carefully what he was going to do. Based on the X-rays and some ultrasound pictures, he was going to take two or three snippets of the suspect tissue and order a frozen section from pathology. This meant that he would send the pieces to the pathology lab and they would freeze them with liquid nitrogen and cut them and look at them right away. If it wasn't cancer, we would know that same day. Regular sections take a day or two to process. He would order those too to make sure.

There was still the chance it was benign. Pam hoped and prayed it was. I hoped and prayed it was. I was still hoping and praying it was two days later as I waited in the lobby of the hospital while Dr. Worchel operated. This was why I had my eyes closed when Dr. Worchel walked up to me and touched my arm. "They think it's cancer," he said.

That was about 12:30. Around 2, they called my name and let me in to see her in a small recovery room. She was still under the influence of the anesthetic. She could barely talk. I wasn't sure she understood what I was saying. When I told her, "Dr. Worchel came up to me and told me, 'They think it's cancer,'" her eyes filled with tears. I tried to wipe them away. More came.

A bossy nurse came in and concluded Pam needed pain medication. She gave her something that made Pam nauseated and gave her chills for several hours. Eventually she felt well enough for me to take her home. She slept a great deal that day and the next.

I went up to school only long enough to run a lab and came back home. Pam was napping. The phone rang. It was Dr. Worchel. He had the permanent section report. It was definitely cancer. Pam woke up and wanted to know what the phone call was about. I told her. She cried some more.

It is good to have regular things to do when a situation like this happens to you. While you are washing a car or cleaning a house, you are doing something familiar that you know how to do. You will succeed. You will finish. At least the car or the house will be better than it was before.

You can say none of these things about dealing with cancer the first time. It is strange. You do not know whether you will succeed. You do not know when the process will be finished, or whether it will finish you. You do not know whether things will be better than before, or ever the same as before, or always worse than before.

So I looked forward to doing ordinary things at this time. We went grocery shopping the following Wednesday. Pam had recovered from the surgery except for a bandage on her sutures. She was standing behind me in line at the checkout counter. I picked up a heavy canned ham from the cart. I tried to put it on the conveyor belt at the cash register. It slipped out of my hand and fell on Pam's right big toe.

She knelt down in pain. I helped her over to a nearby wall. She sat down on the floor and held her toe and rocked back and forth.

People started to stare. I said in my loudest lecture-room voice, "I dropped a can of ham on her *toe!*" That satisfied them. In a few minutes she could stand up again. We went home.

Chapter 7

Sacred Harps

That same week a friend of mine had told me about a Sacred Harp sing that was being held Saturday in a small church in the countryside southeast of San Marcos. Partly to distract ourselves from sitting around the house worrying, we made plans to go.

The Primitive Baptist Church in McMahon, Texas, was founded in 1852. That is only seven years after Texas became a state. In 1900, the church hosted its first annual Sacred Harp sing. The one we attended was therefore the 102nd Sacred Harp sing held at the church.

Here is how a Sacred Harp sing goes. The singers, usually between twenty and fifty of them, arrange their chairs around an empty square, sopranos on one side, tenors, altos, and bases on the other three sides. Each singer holds a Sacred Harp hymnal, a thick book wider than it is high and filled with pages of numbered shape-note hymns. I knew a little about shape-note singing because one of my grandmothers belonged to the Church of Christ, which prohibits the use of musical instruments in its services. Their reasoning is that the New Testament mentions no musical instruments in its descriptions of early Christian worship, so a church wanting to adhere to the literal meaning of Scripture had better not use any either. Shape notes were introduced in the 19th century to help people learn to read music. Each line on the staff has a characteristic note shape associated with it. Since *a cappella* singing was the only kind of music Church of Christers could enjoy in church, they decided to use shape notes.

At the Sacred Harp sing, song leaders stood up in rotation in the center of the square and called out the number of a song. The leader played a pitch pipe for the first note and then commenced to beat time with an arm motion that resembled a person pumping an old-fashioned water well pump. The first time through, the singers sang the notes instead of the words: "so-so-so-la-re-re-re." Then they sang all the verses of the song, quite loudly, with no modulation whatsoever. At first the sound of dozens of full-volume voices seems harsh and chaotic, but soon a strange kind of structure and beauty emerges, unlike any other type of music I have heard.

Some of the songs were very old. One commemorated the death of President Washington. It was probably written not long after the fact. Others were composed as recently as the 1920s. The singing made me feel that I was standing on a high mountain with thousands of people from all ages and walks of life as we beheld the end of the world and the beginning of something that cannot be expressed in words. But Sacred Harp singing comes close to expressing it. Something keeps small crowds of people coming to Sacred Harp sings all over the United States, month after month, year after year, learning the songs from their parents and teaching them to their children.

In the presence of that music, it was not possible to think about the things that Pam and I were going through in the way we thought of them at home in the living room by ourselves. The singers sang of sickness and death, heartbreak and tears. But they kept on singing. At the end of each song there was no applause and no critical comments. Once or twice we heard the leader murmur a quiet, "Good." Then the next leader came up, called out her number, and the next song began.

After a couple of hours, they declared a break. We decided to head home. We had parked in the grass off of the highway. A young man was standing next to our car. He looked as though he wanted to speak to us. It turned out his battery was dead. He wanted to know if we had any jumper cables. We did. I opened the hood of our car and connected up the cables. We tried to start his car for ten or fifteen minutes. It never started. We apologized to him and drove back to San Marcos.

In town, we stopped at a video store. When we came out of the store, *our* car wouldn't start. I tried to push it to get it rolling fast enough to turn the engine over. A Hispanic woman saw me and offered her car and jumper cables. I accepted. We got our car started and drove the rest of the way home.

Chapter 8

In The Shop

The following Tuesday, we went to see Dr. Worchel again. As he described what was going to happen next, I began to understand how doctors work together. They don't.

It is more like an old roundhouse that railroads used to use to repair steam locomotives. A roundhouse was a way to put a number of specialized repair shops in a small area. It was built around a section of track on a turntable that was just long enough for a locomotive to fit on. The engineer would run the locomotive onto the turntable. The turntable then turned to point the track at whichever shop the locomotive needed repairs in: the boiler shop, the valve shop, the firebox shop, the electrical shop, or what have you. The engineer ran the locomotive into the first shop, got the first problem taken care of, backed his engine out onto the turntable, and then moved it to the next shop and so on, until all the repairs were done.

A cancer patient is like the locomotive on the turntable. She is at the center of a radiating network of specialists: oncologists, surgeons, radiologists, anesthesiologists, pathologists, and other specialists. The shops in the roundhouse stood apart from each other, and the locomotive went to one after the other. The cancer patient goes to one specialist after another. The specialists may communicate with each other, usually by faxes from one office to another office. Somehow I had started out with the idea that all the doctors would get together and hold a meeting to discuss her case. This never happened. Apparently, the only time doctors meet together is at business meetings, conventions, and parties. It is the way the system works.

Since the system works this way, the only person who is in a position to know what is really going on at all times is the patient, or someone close to the patient. Pam is a very organized person. She realized quickly that if anyone was going to have a centralized file of all the tests, bills, and other paperwork that her treatment was generating, it had to be her. She bought a large three-ring notebook and began to put the documents in it. I began to take careful notes during appointments and summarized them later for filing. We were glad we did this on more than one occasion. If she had not been so organized, I would have had to do it all myself. But someone needed to do it. The system was not going to do it for us.

I did not understand all of this until several months later. But as Dr. Worchel explained what he thought we should do next, the outlines began to appear in my mind.

First, he told us what the pathology report said, in English. Pam had invasive cancer, meaning it had gone beyond the milk ducts where it probably started and invaded tissues where it didn't belong. But it was "low-grade." That meant that it wasn't as fast-growing as some types of cancer. Still, it was cancer.

It had to come out. The only question was how. Dr. Worchel said that we should see a radiation oncologist and a medical oncologist. Radiation oncologists treat cancer with radiation, and medical oncologists treat it with chemotherapy. The size of the tumor was important. It was probably a little under an inch in diameter. That made it almost too large to do what laymen call a "lumpectomy." In this procedure, the surgeon cuts out the tumor and enough surrounding tissue to make sure that he gets all the cancer that can be detected. The way he tells is to send the parts he cuts out to the pathologist. The pathologist stains them and slices them up to tell whether there are margins of normal cells all around the cancer. If there are, the surgeon got all the cancer he could.

After a lumpectomy, most people receive radiation to kill whatever may be left behind. Radiation can be aimed at the spot where the cancer used to be. Often with small cancers, a lumpectomy and radiation are all that is needed.

Sometimes the tumor is so large in comparison to the breast that taking out only the tumor is not easy or possible. Then the surgeon will perform a mastectomy. He removes all the breast tissue. The woman can choose to use a prosthesis (a fake breast), in which case the doctor simply closes the wound and leaves her flat on that side. Or she can choose to have reconstructive surgery, which involves placing an implant near the space vacated by the breast tissue.

It was too early to make choices. We needed more information. So we made an appointment two days later to see Dr. Timothy Dziuk. (We called his office and were told it rhymes with juke.) We found him in the list of providers in Pam's health plan book. The health plan would pay full price only for services by professionals in their network, so we limited our choices to those who were in the book. If we had had no health insurance, or only the use-once-and-discard type we bought the year before, I do not know what we would have done.

Medical offices cluster around hospitals. Pam's biopsy had taken place at South Austin Hospital, across the street from Dr. Worchel's office. Dr. Dziuk's office was a block up the street from Dr. Worchel's office, in a cancer center building. On the ground floor there was a large, expensive-looking suite that led to some eight or ten doctor's offices and labs. We gave our name and waited. And waited.

A cancer center's waiting room is different than the waiting room of a general practitioner. You will see more seriously ill people there: people using walkers, people carrying oxygen tanks around with them, extremely thin people, and people who are either bald as billiard balls (men), or wear scarves, wigs, or extremely short haircuts (women). We once saw a pleasant-looking woman in late middle age whose right arm from her shoulder to her elbow was swelled to the size of a football. Later we found this is a one of the possible side effects of breast cancer surgery called lymphedema, caused when the circulation of the intercellular fluid called lymph is interrupted. The wait did not make for an encouraging twenty minutes.

Finally they called Pam's name. I went in with her. A nurse weighed Pam and took her blood pressure. Then we went into an examining room and met Dr. Dziuk.

Of all the medical personnel we met during Pam's adventures, I liked Dr. Dziuk the best. It turned out he didn't do a thing to her. That may be one reason I liked him so much.

Dr. Dziuk wore a ring with a fish symbol on it and an interested, confident expression. He pulled out a piece of paper and began to draw pictures. One showed the cancer (he called it "the bad cells") surrounded by normal cells. He said no one knows why cancer starts when or where it does. Sometimes it starts in one location and just grows there for a while, and then spreads out from there. Other times they will open up someone and find lots of little isolated cancers, each surrounded by normal tissue, like scattered wildflowers in a field. Each cancer would appear to have arisen independently of the others. This was called the field effect. I didn't like hearing about that.

However the cancer arose, his specialty was directing radiation at it so as to interrupt the growth cycle. Both normal and cancer cells take a certain time to grow, divide, and grow again. Radiation treatment is timed so that just when a batch of cancer cells is ready to divide, they get blasted by radiation and tend to die at their most vulnerable time. The faster the cells grow, the more vulnerable they are to radiation, which is why radiation can shrink or eradicate many cancers, which grow faster than normal cells.

If Pam decided to have a lumpectomy and it was successful, Dr. Dziuk would be happy to zap her in this calculated fashion to get rid of any remaining cells. Of course, there were no guarantees. He cited statistics that were encouraging about five-year survival rates. I tried to write them down. It was the first time anyone had even indirectly addressed the question, "How long will Pam live?"

We thanked him and left feeling better. I began to take notice of a physician's manner or aura as well as the content of what he had to say. Dr. Dziuk had a great aura. I thought he would be a good guy to play golf with, if I played golf.

When we went back to talk with Dr. Worchel, he asked us to ask Dr. Dziuk what he (Dziuk) would do if Dr. Worchel did a lumpectomy. So we did. (One shop doesn't talk directly to another; the locomotive backs out onto the turntable and goes to the next shop.) Dr. Dziuk gave us a four-part answer that I summarized as follows. There were likely two kinds of cancer going on: invasive (the worse kind), and the less aggressive "ductal carcinoma in situ" or DCIS, which is a kind that grows in the milk ducts but doesn't spread outside them. What Dr. Dziuk said he would do depended on what kind of cancer, if any, was left at the margins of the lump that Dr. Worchel removed. If there were cancer cells at the edges, meaning that some cells were still in Pam, that is called "positive margins." Otherwise it is called "negative margins."

If the margins were negative for both invasive and DCIS, Dr. Dziuk would use radiation.

If the margins were positive for invasive and negative for DCIS, he would consider using radiation.

If the margins were positive for DCIS and negative for invasive, he would recommend a mastectomy.

If the margins were positive for both DCIS and invasive, he would recommend a mastectomy.

We went back to Dr. Worchel with this information. It was clear to me that Dr. Worchel slightly favored the mastectomy because it was more likely to get everything done at once. Pam wanted to think about it some more. We also received the news that the cancer was positive for estrogen receptors, which Dr. Worchel said was good. She finally decided to get a third opinion, so we picked a doctor out of the book that I will call Dr. Smith.

Dr. Smith was a medical oncologist in the same suite as Dr. Dziuk. He was a large, hearty guy with an air of studied casualness. He grabbed Pam's charts and studied them as he talked, asking questions here and there. At the end he said either mastectomy or lumpectomy with radiation were both reasonable choices. It was up to us.

Pam pondered for another few days. Then she called Dr.

Worchel's office and set up an appointment for a lumpectomy on May 9.

Chapter 9

The Lumpectomy

Dr. Worchel had told us about Dr. Susan Love's *Breast Book*. We bought a copy. It is 500 pages of the latest scientific advice and information on the breast, including but not limited to breast cancer. On one page she shows a chart that gives the five-year survival rate for people with various degrees of breast cancer, assuming they are treated properly.

Doctors often talk of stages of cancer. Stage One is the earliest form that is detectible. Stage Four is what you have just before you die of it. According to what we now knew, based upon size and type, Pam's was between Stage One and Stage Two. According to the chart, the five-year survival rate was about 85%. That was more or less what some of the doctors had told us.

I thought about that. My mother, who received only a radical mastectomy and no other treatment until the cancer returned eight years later, was in the 85 percent who survived for at least five years after diagnosis. My father, whose five-year survival rate would have been about 15 percent, died a year after diagnosis. I reminded myself that the five-year survival rate for any randomly selected 100 women of my wife's age (she was 46) was less than 100 percent. I am not an actuary, but probably at least one or two out of every 100 46-year-old women in the U. S. die of various things before they reach their 51st birthday. 85 percent was not 99 percent, but it wasn't 50 percent or 5 percent either.

One thing the lumpectomy would tell us is the state of Pam's lymph nodes. The lymphatic system is a little like the storm drains of the body. Any fluid that seeps outside the blood vessels eventually winds up as lymph in the lymph vessels. These drain into concentrations of antibody cells in lymph nodes. The lymph nodes under the arm are one of the first places that breast cancer cells spread to when they start spreading beyond the breast. So surgeons routinely remove certain lymph nodes on the affected side whenever they do a lumpectomy. They call this "axillary dissection."

One way they have developed to figure out which nodes to take out is called a "sentinel node biopsy." The surgeon injects a blue dye at the location of the tumor. He then has seven minutes to look for the nodes under the arm that have received the dye. Those are the ones that are most likely to have harbored any cancer cells that spread. Dr. Worchel planned to do this when he did the lumpectomy. The results would place Pam in a more specific part of the survival chart. If the cancer had not yet spread to any of the lymph nodes, it would be better than if it had. I thought of the time when I wanted to know if our toilet tank had a slow leak. I dropped some blue food coloring in the tank and waited to see if any showed up in the bowl.

May 9 was a Thursday. Dr. Worchel told us that Pam might have to stay overnight, so Wednesday night she packed a small suitcase. The semester was over, so I was free to accompany her. I was glad that my job allowed me enough free time to take Pam to her appointments and to be with her during the surgery.

Teaching looks easy. If you looked at my schedule for the spring, it said that I must be in class for four hours of lecturing and four hours of laboratories every week, plus five office hours. I also did some research, but when I did it was up to me. I know some teachers who do things completely unrelated to teaching with all the time that they do not spend actually in the classroom. Generally they are not good teachers. I was also glad that I spent fifteen or twenty hours a week the previous summer preparing lectures for the following year. That freed me up to spend time with Pam when I needed to.

After we checked in at the hospital admission desk, the first order of business was something called a lymphoscintigraphy. In order to have an idea of what was going on with the lymph nodes, Dr. Worchel set up this procedure.

It works this way. The radiologist injects into the tumor a small amount of technetium, which is an artificial radioactive element. Then every half hour or so for the next two hours, she positions a detector over the patient and profiles where the technetium has gone. Usually it goes into the lymph nodes that receive drainage from the tumor site. The radiologist marks the skin above the location where the lymph nodes are to guide the surgeon.

Pam was in the nuclear medicine suite off and on from about 8:30 to nearly 11. When she came out the first time, she told me what had happened. The radiologist tried to use an ultrasound machine to find the tumor. She couldn't. She got some help from two or three other technicians, and they couldn't find it either. Finally Pam said, "If you want me to find it for you, I can show you where it is." She rolled over further (she was lying on a special narrow table) and pointed at a spot. Then they found it, did the injection, and waited.

While we were waiting between scans, Pam was free to come out and sit with me down the hallway from the nuclear medicine room. At one point, we heard a crash, a couple of screams and moans, and some scrambling in there. Later, Pam found out that they had tried to scan a semiconscious man. He fell off the narrow table on top of the radiologist, and it took four people to get him up.

At 11:30, they took us into one of the small preparatory rooms that you go into before surgery. There was a hospital bed, an easy chair, and some medical equipment in each one. Pam changed into a hospital johnny open at the back. A nurse came with a wheelchair, Pam got into it, and she wheeled Pam away.

I did not bring Shakespeare with me this time. I decided to pray instead. I prayed that the nodes would be free of cancer and that the margins would be clear (or negative). I found a comfortable chair in the hospital lobby and sat there with my eyes closed.

You may not be able to imagine how anyone can pray for the same thing for more than a few minutes. It helps if you believe it will do some good. At the time, it was the best way I believed I could help.

I knew nothing about surgery. I cannot stand the sight of blood. I look the other way when I get a shot in my arm. I would be worse than useless in an operating room. But I could sit there and pray that Dr. Worchel and everyone around him knows their business and does it as well as it can be done. Many things can go wrong in an operating room. I didn't want any of them to go wrong when Pam was involved. If I were a doctor, I am sure that I could have prayed more intelligently. But God knows more than any doctor.

In the middle of all this, my cell phone rang. It was the pastor of the church we used to attend in Massachusetts. His name is ThankGod Maduka. He and his wife are from Nigeria. The woman named Ginger who prayed for Pam before her not-biopsy eight years earlier was from their church. They have kept up with us and prayed with us over the phone several times since they heard the news about Pam. Pastor Maduka was calling from his job. I told him things were going well as far as I knew, but to keep praying. He said that he would. I thanked him for calling.

I prayed some more. The phone rang again. It was a friend of Pam's from work I shall call Tammy Martin. I said more or less the same things to Tammy that I said to Pastor Maduka. Tammy herself is an answer to prayer. At Pam's job in Massachusetts, she had no close friends. When we came down to Texas, I prayed that she would get a Christian friend at work. I prayed this regularly for months. Nothing happened at first. Pam met Tammy shortly after she began working here, and to make a long and complicated story short, Tammy became a Christian, and Pam's best friend at work.

Around 2, Dr. Worchel walked up to me, still in his green operating outfit. He said that things went reasonably well. He felt pretty good about the sentinel node biopsy. He was able to find the ones stained with blue dye and got several. But his face changed expression when he talked about the lumpectomy. He got all he could see, but there was a lot of scar tissue from the biopsy under the nipple. He didn't want to talk about that much. He said that Pam would be out of the recovery room in about an hour. I thanked him and he left.

The hospital loaned me a beeper to carry so they could let me know when Pam was ready for me to see her. Three o'clock came and went. At 3:30 I decided to ask someone to see what was going on. I did not want to be a pest and nag the desk nurse every ten minutes. But busy medical staff people tend to deal with things that obviously need attention: incoming ambulance patients, irate family members, and other attention-getting things. If you just stand in the background and assume you will come to their minds at the right time, you will sometimes be mistaken.

When I asked, they told me that when Pam was ready, they would send her straight up to her room. This was the first time I heard anything about a room. I went over to the outpatient desk and a young woman told me what room Pam would be taken to. It was on the fourth floor.

I rode the elevator to the fourth floor and went down the hall to the room. It was a double. Someone was in the bed next to the hallway. I decided to wait in the hall. I waited for half an hour.

Finally, here came Pam in a stretcher. She looked weak and greenish. She couldn't talk very well. The orderly helped her get into the bed next to the window. She dozed off and on and said she felt nauseated. She managed to suck on a piece of ice I gave her. When supper came about 5:30, she ate a piece of bread.

Dr. Worchel showed up shortly after that. He explained that the pathology report on the lumpectomy would be available in a day or two. The results of the axillary dissection (the lymph nodes) will take longer. The hope was that the lump's margins were clear and that there was no cancer in the lymph nodes.

I stayed with Pam overnight that night. The only living things at our house besides us were a cat and some potted plants, all of which could take care of themselves for a day or two. If I had gone home I would have just stayed up all night worrying about how Pam was doing. So I stayed. The cell phone rang some more: my sister in Fort Worth, another friend at Pam's work, another church friend. I told them Pam was doing as well as could be expected.

There was a kind of lounge chair next to the bed. It tilted back but did not flatten out. I decided that it would have to do. The window overlooked a flat roof and the Austin neighborhood near the hospital. It got dark around seven.

The woman next to us kept the television on. Around 9 I pulled a blanket over myself and tried to sleep. Instead I watched most of "Stuart Little" on the TV. The woman turned it off around 11.

At midnight, a nurse came in to check Pam's blood pressure. She used a little machine that made just enough noise to wake me up.

At four A. M., it was time for another blood-pressure check. I watched this one too.

At six, I decided to look for something to eat. I found a nest of vending machines down the hall and bought some cookies.

An orderly brought Pam's breakfast at 7:30. Pam's appetite was better. She was attached to an IV on a pole, which she wheeled into the bathroom with her.

At 9:30, Dr. Worchel appeared. He heard from the pathology people already. "Good news and bad news: your nodes are clear, far as they can tell, but the margins were positive." This meant a mastectomy. He talked about scheduling a visit to a plastic surgeon. They are among the hardest kind of specialists to see. He also mentioned that there was another axillary node test for micrometastases that would come back later next week. We thanked him and he left.

Pam expressed a strong desire to go home. Dr. Worchel said she was ready and he would issue the order. In another hour or so, a nurse came by and took out Pam's IV. After that, I just picked up our bags and we split for home. I had a semi-conscious awareness that we were probably skipping some kind of paperwork, but both of us just wanted out of there.

When we got home, there was a message on the answering machine. It was a floor nurse who said we should have signed the release papers and got some instructions before we left. She wanted us to call back.

First Pam had to cry. She wanted to know why, with all these people praying that her margins would be clear, that they weren't? I could not tell her.

Chapter 10

Take Your Choice

In the days that followed, we talked about what to do. The more Pam thought about it, the more she thought reconstruction was something she wanted to have. "I want something positive to come out of the next surgery," she said. We had not talked with a plastic surgeon yet. Dr. Worchel recommended a person I shall call Dr. Carlson. Pam made an appointment with him for May 17. The day before we went, we got a call from Dr. Worchel's office. The test for micrometastases was negative. Her nodes had no cancer. This was good news. I looked in the *Breast Book* for the category that includes people with Pam's type of cancer and no lymph nodes involved. The five-year survival rate is 95%.

Dr. Carlson's office looked very different than Dr. Worchel's office. Dr. Worchel's office was small and brightly lit. The only decorations were a photograph of a mother mountain lion carrying her cub in her mouth and a framed poem to the effect that "M. D." means "My Daddy." On the other hand, Dr. Carlson's waiting room was the size of an average living room. It had deep pile carpet, antique tables and cabinets, and wood paneling of a kind I have seen only in the offices of expensive lawyers or in old photographs of Victorian men's clubs.

Pam gave her name to one of the women behind the counter.

The woman was dressed and made up as if she were serving customers at an elegant women's clothing store. We sat down and waited. I looked at the other couples in the room. I wondered who among the other women was here because she had to be, and who was here because she wanted to be.

Another young woman appeared at the door and called Pam's name. We followed her down a long hall, around a corner, and into a large examining room with a fancy motorized chair in it. The woman handed Pam a silk Halston nightgown and asked her to take off her top before Dr. Carlson came. Pam told me that Halston gowns are the height of fashion. I said, "Fine." She went behind a curtain in the corner of the room and changed.

While we waited, I noted from diplomas on the wall that Dr. Carlson obtained his undergraduate degree from Harvard in biology. Then he went to Baylor for his medical training. That was about twenty years ago.

The door opened. It was Dr. Carlson. He had short curly black hair, an even tan, and a smooth manner of speaking. When he asked Pam a question, she spouted a bunch of medical terminology about her condition. He listened. When she finished, he said that the goal of the surgery is "symmetrical breasts." He asked Pam to take off her gown.

I was in the examining room when Dr. Worchel examined Pam in this way. It took some getting used to. But I knew Dr. Worchel's interest in the situation was purely technical. It didn't bother me that much. Dr. Carlson's interest was partly technical and partly esthetic. The technical part did not bother me. But the esthetic part did. I kept my mouth shut and watched.

Dr. Carlson explained that there are basically four ways to reconstruct a breast after a mastectomy. The first way is to put an implant directly into the space left by the missing breast. (This is what the surgeons did to my mother after her mastectomy.) He doesn't do this anymore because "it doesn't work." The implant never attains a natural shape. The skin over it can easily become necrotic. ("Necrotic" is doctor's talk for "dead.") This is also what happened to my mother.

The second way is to create a pocket behind the muscle wall that is behind the missing breast. During the same surgery as the mastectomy, he inserts a temporary implant in this pocket. It is a silicone bag with a kind of valve and a magnet that helps the doctor find the valve under the skin. Over a period of four to six weeks, he inserts more saline solution into the bag so that the muscles and other tissues gradually accommodate themselves to the increasing size of the implant. Once this is done, he performs a second surgery to replace the temporary implant with the permanent one. "Permanent" is a manner of speaking. He told us that the failure rate is about 1% per year.

The third way involves removing a slice of fatty tissue from the patient's back and using it to replace part of what is missing, and making up the difference with an implant. This involves considerable more recovery time than the second way. It also requires the removal of healthy tissue.

The fourth way is to take fat and a muscle from the stomach area and use it to replace all the missing breast tissue. There are no implants involved here. But it takes six to eight weeks to recover from this one.

After he examined Pam, he said that she was a candidate for any of the three kinds of this surgery that he did. I was expecting a sales pitch for one or the other, but he did nothing of the kind.

The next step was to take pictures. Right next to the examining room there was a specialized photography studio. Dr. Carlson said his assistants would take the pictures, and then Pam could think a few days about what she wanted to do. Then the same young woman as before came in and handed Pam what she called "photo panties." It was basically a paper thong. They took a picture of her head only, and then the rest separately. I understood the legal reasons for doing this. But it didn't make me feel any better about it. I continued to keep my mouth shut. But it was hard not to laugh when the woman said "photo panties."

I stayed in the examining room while Pam got her pictures taken. I had no desire to watch the process.

In a few moments Pam came back and put on her clothes. The

young woman told us to meet her in the library down the hall. The library was one of the more pleasant rooms in the large office suite. Its windows looked out on North Austin, with a particularly fine view of the roof of a brake-repair shop on Lamar.

In the library, Pam was presented with a large photo album that showed the before-and-after results of the various kinds of surgery Dr. Carlson does in these cases. After the young woman left us to ourselves, Pam asked me if I wanted to look.

In the seventh chapter of the letter to the Romans, St. Paul talks about his fleshly nature and his spiritual nature. This is not the same thing as body and spirit. We are embodied spirits as long as we live. Everything we do on earth involves both body and spirit. He also calls the fleshly nature the "old man." He means the way he was before he met Christ.

The old man did not die all at once when he met Christ, and it is the same with me. That old man very much wanted to see the pictures. But not for the reason of helping Pam to decide what method of surgery to use. The new man wanted Pam to have the freedom to select anything or nothing. He knew that Pam wanted to have a body that pleases him.

After taking these things into consideration, I told Pam I did not want to see the pictures. So I stood at the window and looked out onto the roof of the brake shop while I heard Pam say, "Ooohh . . . . mmm.. . . . .So that's it . . . .oh, gee . . . ."

Finally she saw enough. As we were on our way out, the women at the front desk asked Pam which way she was leaning. The way they asked reminded me of car salesmen. Normally I let Pam speak for herself, but that time I told them that she was standing absolutely straight right now.

Chapter 11

Chemo Ahead

In the fourth week of May we went to see Dr. Dziuk and Dr. Smith again. By that time they had both received the pathology reports from the lumpectomy and the axillary dissection (the lymph nodes). Dr. Dziuk, the radiologist, said that he was recommending a mastectomy because the margins were not clear. This is just what he told us he would tell us before. He said there were individual cancer cells in the material they removed as well as strings of them. This led him to suspect there might be some cancer throughout the breast. His radiation was too focused to do much good in that case. That was why mastectomy was the best choice.

The appointment with the medical oncologist, Dr. Smith, was set up for right after the appointment with Dr. Dziuk. As we left Dr. Dziuk's office, I looked at Pam. She was holding herself together. But it was not easy for her. It was hard for her to let go of the idea of keeping her breast.

In the twenty-five years that we have been married, Pam let her hair grow for about twenty of them. Her hair was a medium blonde with no gray at all, even at the age of forty-six. When it got below her waist, she would occasionally have the ends trimmed. But for most of the last twenty years it has been about three feet long. When she let it down it was one of her most attractive features. She spent fifteen or twenty minutes every day combing it and braiding it.

That is why one of the things she feared most was having to undergo chemotherapy. We knew generally that most kinds of chemotherapy for breast cancer cause you to lose your hair.

We waited a suitable time, were admitted into one of Dr. Smith's examining rooms, and waited some more. Eventually Dr. Smith knocked on the examining-room door and opened it. His own hair is wavy and gray. I decide this time that he looked like a stockbroker who played golf a lot. He started off the conversation by congratulating Pam on having clear nodes (no cancer in them). Then he got down to business.

He explained that if Pam were eighty years old, he would not recommend chemotherapy. He did not have to say the reason, which was that the chances are she would die of something else before the cancer came back. I had a great aunt in Fort Worth who had been through the same situation with breast cancer in the last year. She was in her seventies, but she had chemo anyway.

"However," he said, "you're young." We had no argument with him there. Therefore, he was recommending chemotherapy.

Pam asked, "The kind where you lose your hair?"

"Afraid so."

She almost cried right there in front of him. But she held herself in.

The kind of chemotherapy he recommended was called "FAC." This stands for three different kinds of chemicals: 5-fluorouracil, Adriamycin, and cyclophosphamide. He said that we should wait a few weeks until she recovered from the effects of the mastectomy, which he assumed would be soon. Then she would get six chemotherapy treatments spaced at three-week intervals. He said he would ask Dr. Worchel to put in a "port" during the mastectomy. This is a thin plastic tube that leads from a kind of receiving chamber implanted under the skin to a large artery near the heart. In that way, the concentrated chemicals do not land in a small artery and burn it up. Instead they get diluted in the high volume of blood in the large artery. I concentrated on this technical detail until the conversation was over.

On the way out, Pam started to cry. I guided her to her car and we sat there while she continued to cry. She wasn't able to stop crying.

She wanted to go home. I had driven up to meet her for the appointments in my car. I decided to leave it there and drive her home in her car. I figured we could get my car back later somehow.

She gradually calmed down during the hour it took to drive from Austin to San Marcos. Then she started to cry again when we got home. I hugged her and handed her tissues. It was a long day.

The next day she stayed home from work. She called Dr. Worchel's office to set up the next surgery date for June 12, about two weeks away. For a long while after the phone call, Pam sat in the bedroom and looked out the window at our bird feeder. She saw a small bird with a bright yellow back, a dark blue head, and a scarlet-red belly. She looked it up in a bird book. It was a painted bunting. She had never seen one before. She told me it was a gorgeous bird.

The following Saturday, she called me to the window again. She said the painted bunting was back. I looked outside and there it was. After that, we didn't see another one for several years.

Chapter 12
Memorial Day

Near the end of May, we went to talk with Dr. Worchel about how the next operation would go. Pam decided on the type of breast reconstruction surgery that involved a tissue expander and a permanent implant afterwards.

This surgery will be more complicated than the lumpectomy.

First, Dr. Worchel will excise all the breast tissue in the left breast. That will not take long, perhaps twenty or thirty minutes. Then he will insert the Passport, the trade name for the type of port that he likes to install when he has the opportunity. Most surgeons these days, he explained, go with the type of port that is installed on the chest and is inserted in a vein near the clavicle, because the surgery is easier. But an arm-mounted port, the type he prefers, is safer for the patient, he said. The surgery is trickier, however. He brought out a plastic model arm with the Passport mounted in a typical location on the fascia under the skin. The arm had a removable section that let you see the port to appreciate its low, sleek profile. He showed us what a port and its attached tube looked like. The port itself was a shiny polished-steel object with a round plastic center. It would look at home hanging on a board in an auto parts store in the custom running lights section.

Next, he went over to where a detailed anatomical chart of the human torso hung on the wall. He twirled the port's catheter tube around his finger as he explained the insertion process. First, he would tie off the distal (farther) part of the arm vein. Then he would insert the tube with a "J-wire" inside it. The J-wire is a thin springy wire that makes the tube rigid enough to go through the vein as the surgeon pushes it in. I thought of the electricians I have seen at construction sites. They build long steel conduit pipes into the walls of buildings for the electrical cables. Then the electricians stick a thing called a fishtape into the conduit and run it inside the smooth walls of the conduit to the junction box. Then they tie the cable to the fishtape and pull the cable through. The J-wire was a fishtape for the port tube.

The J-wire also helps the surgeon see where the tube is going as he guides it up the arm, past the shoulder, and into the chest area. During this part of the procedure, assistants bring a portable fluoroscope (an X-ray machine) into the operating room so the surgeon can see where the J-wire (and the tube) is at all times. The tube by itself would not show up on a fluoroscope.

There are several things that can go wrong. Dr. Worchel explained that he was legally obliged to tell us about them. For one thing, the J-wire can take a wrong turn and go into the lung, causing hemorrhaging and lung damage. For another thing, it can go too far past the large vein leading to the heart and into the heart itself, damaging the heart. "You can die," he said, if that happens. But he takes things carefully and slowly and rarely has any problems. If he runs into signs of trouble, he will simply back everything out and try again.

He took a look at Pam and said, "You're nice and skinny. I don't think I'll have much trouble with you."

Once the tube is in its proper place, he will remove the J-wire and attach the tube to the metal port. Then he will sew the port onto the fascia with two stitches, stitch the skin closed over the port, and call in Dr. Carlson. The surgery will have taken about an hour and a half so far.

Dr. Carlson will then take over. He will insert the temporary tissue expander through the chest incision left by Dr. Worchel.

There is considerable pulling and tugging involved, but Dr. Carlson did not go into the detail that Dr. Worchel did with us. Once Dr. Carlson is finished, the operation will be over.

We thanked Dr. Worchel and left. I was glad all that was not being done to me.

The following Saturday began Memorial Day weekend. We decided to drive up to Fort Worth to visit some of my relatives. Besides my sister, I have several aunts and cousins there. My last blood-relative uncle lived in Fort Worth and was buried on the day I began my job at the university in San Marcos, in September of 2000. He was a much-decorated Air Force pilot who flew during World War II, the Korean War, and the Vietnam War. He outlived my father and their brother. All three smoked and all three eventually died of lung cancer. The Air Force uncle was named Leonard Perry Stephan.

When we got to Fort Worth, Uncle Perry's widow, Aunt Percy, invited us to go with her and her daughter Ann Marsh to the Memorial Day ceremonies at the new veteran's cemetery in Grand Prairie. No one calls the daughter by her real name. She is Marcie to everyone who knows her. After a brief marriage that ended in divorce, Marcie turned from a wild teenager to one of the most dependable persons in that branch of the family. She has either taught school or been a school counselor for fifteen years or more. She agreed to lead us out to the cemetery, which we have never seen before. She got in her Buick and zoomed down the freeway. It was hard to keep up with her in our Jetta, but I managed.

The cemetery was built on some land that was once part of a naval air station. We drove by a long line of American flags near a bandstand that was set up on the shores of a pond, and parked in a grassy area some distance away. It was hot and sunny. I wondered whether Aunt Percy could walk the distance. In the last three years, her husband had died of lung cancer after years of emphysema, she had had breast cancer, a mastectomy, and chemotherapy. If she has endured all that, I thought, she can probably take a little sun. She got out of the car and plunged along so fast that the rest of us had to hurry to keep up.

We found a spot on the grassy hill between the bandstand and the row of flags. Percy sat down on the ground. We followed her example. I wished I had a hat. The band played military music. A politician made a speech. Another politician made another speech. I dozed off in the sun. My wife saw me dozing and touched the back of my hand with a cold bottle of water. I woke up with a giant twitch. The women around me all laughed. The speeches ended. We got up and walked back to the car.

Percy said we would stop by Perry's grave on the way out. We pulled in behind them and walked the dozen or so feet from the curb to the gravesite. His grave is at the front of a row. He was seventy-nine when he died. World War II veterans were dying so fast that they were lucky to get a half-hour slot in the cemetery schedule on a Tuesday for the funeral. Other families walked up to other markers, read, chatted, and placed flowers on the graves.

After a few minutes, we said good-bye to Percy and Marcie, got back in our car, and drove back to San Marcos. We were pretty quiet along the way.

Chapter 13
Mastectomy And Reconstruction

Pam's next surgery was scheduled for a Wednesday in the middle of June. Surgeons like to operate either at the crack of dawn or right after lunch. This was an after-lunch surgery. On the day of the surgery, Pam didn't eat lunch, because the hospital requires the patient to fast after midnight the day before. I stayed home with her in the morning. She was nervous and cried some. Once we got in the car and began to do something, she got better.

This surgery was set up at a different hospital than the one where Pam had her failed lumpectomy, mainly because Dr. Carlson prefers this one. When the anesthesiologist came by to chat with us in the little pre-op room, Pam explained to him the nausea problems she had with the previous anesthetic. He said he would give her some pills and special medication to prevent that. After he left, we chatted about nothing in particular. Finally the time came. They took her away and I went to the waiting room. I was told to expect that the surgery may take up to four hours.

In a short while, the pastor from our church and his wife showed up. We talked, went into the hospital chapel to pray, and wound up in the coffee shop talking again for most of the time. Father Len is a former Catholic priest who decided to marry. This had a decided effect on his career: "At that point," he says, "the

Catholic Church informed me they no longer needed my services."
He got married to Nancy and eventually became the pastor of a small
Anglican church.

He didn't talk about that during Pam's surgery. Instead, he told
funny stories about the time he was invited to substitute for another
pastor on a small Caribbean island one summer. This ideal
Caribbean vacation was not all it was advertised to be. Next, Larry,
the husband of a woman at church who had a mastectomy six years
ago showed up. He was a sales representative at a TV station in Fort
Worth where my mother worked for a brief time when I was about
seven. I vaguely recalled some very positive memories of that time.
He told a story about the time he was in the station lobby one day
and saw Bing Crosby and Ben Hogan go through. They were
thinking about buying the station. We talked about anything and
everything but surgery.

A little before two o'clock, Dr. Worchel appeared. He was
wearing the same kind of green scrubs I saw him in after the last
surgery. They have the name of his favorite hospital stitched on
them, which isn't the hospital we're in. He said that everything went
fine with his part, and now Dr. Carlson was doing his bit. I thanked
him and he headed off down the hall. I went back to talk with Father
Len and Nancy some more. Larry excused himself after a while.

Around three, Nancy suggested that we head back to the waiting
area in case they wanted to find me again. As we arrived, Dr. Carlson
came up to me and said that everything went fine with his part too.
He was wearing a new-looking set of scrubs with his initials
monogrammed on the pocket. He left promptly. I kept on waiting.
After they heard from the surgeon, Father Len and Nancy said good-
bye. Now it was just me and Isaiah, which I was reading when I
wasn't praying.

At 6:30, the staff people chased everyone out of the day-surgery
waiting room. We went upstairs to the overnight waiting room. It
was less crowded but felt less hospitable. There was less furniture
and more TVs. I discovered that it was hard to read Isaiah against a
background of "Wheel of Fortune."

At 7:15, an old man volunteering at a desk called me up and

gave me a room number. I took the elevator and found the room. There was no one in the room but Kelle, a nurse who was preparing the bed for Pam. Kelle asked me how Pam found her lump. Her own mother and aunt had the disease. She makes a point of asking how each breast cancer patient discovered her problem. It struck me that Kelle was not simply doing a job.

This hospital is a Catholic hospital. There are crucifixes on the walls here and there. The equipment is not as uniformly new-looking as it was in the first hospital. But the people at this hospital seem to be more interested in the patients.

In a few minutes an orderly wheeled Pam in on a gurney. She looked sleepy but not green at all. The orderly and Kelle got her into bed. She dozed the rest of the evening. It was a private room, so there was no TV to contend with. I arranged myself on the lounge chair next to the bed, covered myself with a blanket, and tried to sleep. I was intermittently successful. But I was awake to witness the 1:30 AM and 4:30 AM blood-pressure checks.

When Pam was awake enough to talk the next day, she told me that she had no nausea at all after this surgery. She was not in much pain. There was a large bandage over the left part of her chest and a small tube leading to a clear plastic object shaped like a hand grenade. This was the drain. A nurse showed Pam how to empty it and squeeze it so as to create a vacuum inside when you hook it back up. That way any fluids are sucked through the tube instead of building up inside to cause swelling. She will keep the drain for a few days.

At one that afternoon, Dr. Worchel showed up to check on Pam. He said she was doing fine. He said he would let us go home later in the day. Dr. Carlson showed up after that and explained some more about the drain. He said he would take it out next week. At four-thirty, the nurse came in and asked us to sign some papers. We followed the rules this time. After that, we were free to go.

Chapter 14

Recovery

Pam stayed home all the rest of the week and into the following week. I was not teaching that summer, so my only scheduled obligations were meetings in Austin once or twice a week for research. I had plenty to do, but I could do most of it at home.

The following Tuesday, Pam developed diarrhea. She drank a lot of fluids, but they kept going right through her. That afternoon, she got weak and light-headed. I called my sister, who said if Pam didn't get better to call Dr. Worchel. She didn't, and I did. I put Pam on the phone. Dr. Worchel asked her a lot of questions. One of the medications she took after surgery was Ceftin, a broad-spectrum antibiotic. It is a very bad thing to develop an infection after surgery, so that is why she received the antibiotic. Ceftin is so powerful that it kills most of the "good" bacteria in the intestinal tract. Without these, the tract cannot work properly. Sometimes this clears the way for a harmful type of bacteria to invade the tract. Dr. Worchel said if she didn't get better soon, we should go to an emergency room and have them check for this problem.

She didn't get any better. That night around nine-thirty, she asked me to take her to the emergency room.

San Marcos has one small hospital. There were not many people in its waiting room that evening. I sat down at a counter in front of a glass panel and gave the receptionist Pam's Blue Cross card and a check for fifty dollars. Someone came and got Pam and took her through a door. They did not invite me to follow.

About an hour later, a tall man clad in blue appeared with a clipboard in his hand. He called out, "Stephan!"

I jumped up and ran to him. He stared at me like I was a Martian. Then he said "Pam?"

"That's my wife."

"I figured it wasn't you. Where is she?"

"The last time I saw her she went through that door there."

"Oh, I saw the clipboard on the rack and thought . . . that's all right. They'll come get you in a while." And he went away.

Eventually I got in to see her. We spent long periods of waiting interrupted once in a while by a nurse or technician with a question or a needle. This went on until half past two in the morning. All they did was to give Pam a can of Gatorade, take some blood samples, and tell her that she did not have the bad kind of infection that Dr. Worchel was worried about. Then they let us go home.

The problem got a little better over the weekend. Pam called Dr. Carlson Monday, who said to take a non-prescription antidiarrheal. It stopped the problem immediately. But dehydration tired her out so much that she felt draggy and tired the rest of the week.

While she stayed home trying to recuperate, several of her friends loaned her videos. We do not watch over-the-air television at home, but we do watch videotaped movies. One of the videos a friend loaned us was produced by Reinhard Bonnke Ministries. Reinhard Bonnke is a German evangelist who preaches mainly in Africa. The video was a well-produced documentary. According to the video, a dead pastor was raised back to life at a church where a Bonnke revival service was going on. The video showed the pastor's death certificate, the rudimentary mortuary where his body was injected with embalming chemicals, the coffin he was laid in, and the wife who prayed that he would come back to life. There are clips of him as he was reviving, and an interview with the pastor himself. He says he received a vision of Heaven and Hell while he was dead.

As I was writing this, I looked on the Internet to see how to spell Bonnke correctly. Reinhard Bonnke Ministries is still in business in Orlando, Florida. There are also several websites that discuss the video at length and try to find faults with it. At several of the Bonnke revival meetings, dozens of people have been crushed to death in crowds. None of these people were raised from the dead, the reports say.

Chapter 15

Haircut

After less than a week, Pam went back to Dr. Carlson, the plastic surgeon, to have the drain removed. He set up an appointment for early July for an expansion treatment. On the same day we saw Dr. Smith.

The expansion treatment went well. Dr. Carlson told her it was the only one she might need. There was not much expansion needed to match the size of the other breast.

Every time we visited a doctor in those days, we brought along a cloth bag that held a large plastic binder with all her medical reports and paperwork in it. I carried it because it was too heavy for her to carry.

We got to the waiting room in the cancer center across the street from the hospital where Dr. Smith has his offices. Pam signed in and we talked about what would happen next. Now that the surgery was done, Dr. Smith would want to start chemotherapy.

After a half hour or so, the receptionist called Pam's name. We went into an area with a nurse's station. One of the nurses weighed Pam and directed us to an examining room. We waited some more. I looked at the objects on the wall. One was a photo of Dr. Smith at some ceremonial event. His hair was black then. Another was a cartoon. It shows a woman talking to a man. Her breasts are squashed flat like pancakes. The caption reads, "Yes, I did have a mammogram today. How did you know?"

Dr. Smith knocked on the door and bustled in. "How is everybody today?" he asked. It turns out that he had not seen the pathology report from the mastectomy yet. Pam brought a copy with her. She handed it to him. He sat and studied it in silence. After a minute or two, he looked up at us and said that he thought the tumor was bigger than we believed at first. "More like 2.5 centimeters than 1.5 centimeters. That's edging into the Stage Two category."

Pam got a grim expression on her face. I saw she was edging close to losing it again. Dr. Smith asked her if she was all right. "I'll be okay," she said.

He said it was just a matter of 2.5 centimeters versus 1.5 centimeters, not that big a deal. He shuffled through some papers in front of him. I asked him about some survival percentages that he had mentioned before. He said he had a good computer program for that. He'd go see if a computer was free. He seemed glad for an excuse to leave the room.

I asked Pam how she was doing. She said she would get through it. But Dr. Smith wasn't helping that much.

When he came back, he said he wasn't able to get on a computer. I asked him what chemotherapy he would recommend. He said six sessions of treatments once every three weeks. Pam was hoping for four.

There wasn't a lot more to say. He said for us to go over and meet the people in the chemotherapy room. We talked about when to start, and I suggested Monday July 29. That would be the day after we got back from a weekend in New England. He said fine.

The chemotherapy room was a pleasant, light-filled area at the corner of the building. We met a nurse with a gentle Scottish accent. She showed us the easy chairs, the little TVs, the bookshelves, and the other fittings inside each therapy space around the perimeter of the room. There were about eight spaces arranged in a ring around a central bench, with a nurse's station on one side of the bench. The nurse explained how things would go. Pam would come in and have an IV inserted. Then they would give her some premedication to make things go better. Then they would give her the three chemicals, each at a different rate. Then as long as she felt all right, she would go home. The whole thing would take about two hours.

"What will happen after that?" Pam asked. "How sick do you typically get?"

"Oh, it varies," said the nurse. She said that with modern anti-nausea drugs, most people may feel slightly tired and draggy for a few days. She might plan on staying home for a day or two after each treatment. But if the treatment was on a Wednesday, she would probably be fine to go back to work the following Monday.

After that, Pam would need to come in once a week to have her blood tested until the next treatment. The chemotherapy attacks rapidly growing cells all over the body, which is why hair usually falls out. The hair-follicle cells and the bone-marrow cells that produce white and red blood cells grow faster than other cells, and are more sensitive than other cells to chemotherapy. Since white blood cells fight infection and red blood cells carry oxygen, it was important to keep tabs on those levels in case they got too low. And if they did, they had modern drugs to boost your levels back up to where they ought to be. So if things went the way they were supposed to, taking chemotherapy would not be much of a problem.

Anything can look easy when you don't have to do it yet. We thanked the nurse and left.

Chemotherapy would almost certainly make Pam go bald. Dr. Smith told us of one patient he had with very dark coarse hair who managed to hold on to hers. But the lighter the hair, the more likely it is to fall out, he said, looking ruefully at Pam's blonde locks.

A week or so later, Pam went to a special wig shop in Austin and bought a wig. She named it Samantha. It was a little lighter than her own hair and shorter than shoulder length. She planned to have her hair cut to match the wig. That way, when she switched to the wig people would be less likely to notice.

When a person learns she has cancer, she has to decide whom to tell. Some people tell no one. Some people tell everyone. Pam realized that the news that someone has cancer is unpleasant for most people to hear. She decided to tell only a few people at her job. She told her boss, who needed to know because Pam wanted to apply for a sick leave pool. She told a few close friends at work. And we told my sister.

Pam did not tell her mother or father. They live in Fort Worth. Her mother has a emotional health disorder. In 1994, she became so difficult to deal with that Pam told her not to contact us any more. Her mother complied. Pam has not spoken to her mother since then. Pam's father gets so much grief from Pam's mother if he does anything she doesn't like, that he has not tried to call us more than once a year. Usually he calls when his wife is in the shower.

So for people who do not know she has cancer, it will appear that she has simply gotten tired of her long hair and cut it in a shorter style. This is how she wants to do things.

The day after we talked with Dr. Smith was the 4th of July. It rained most of the day. I took out Susan Love's *Breast Book* and tried to explain to Pam about the survival percentages that we asked Dr. Smith about. Afterward, Pam said that she wished Dr. Smith had done as good a job as I had.

The Wednesday after the 4th, Pam got her hair cut. She tried to prepare me for the loss of her hair by buying some software called Cosmo Makeover. You scan a picture of your face, put it in the software, and it lets you try on all kinds of virtual wigs, makeup, and other facial modifications. Pam took some of the more outlandish fright-wig-looking things and put them around her face. Then she posted the results on a website and sent the URL to another artistic woman at her job. The lady thought it was a scream.

When she came back from the hairdresser's with short hair, I told her it made her look younger. I wasn't saying that just to be nice. Other people told her the same thing. She decided to donate her long hair to an organization called Locks of Love, which uses it to make wigs for children with cancer.

Chapter 16

A Little Bit of Nigeria

On the last weekend of July, Pam flew up to meet me in New England, where I had flown earlier in the week on business. After sixteen years of living in western Massachusetts, we still had more friends there than we had made so far in San Marcos. We planned this trip back in May. Pastor ThankGod had told us that he and his wife Julie were planning a party on the weekend of our visit to celebrate their twenty-fifth wedding anniversary. They invited us to come.

ThankGod and Julie are Nigerians. In the 1960s, Nigeria went through a civil war and internal conflicts. Many thousands of Nigerians died at the hands of other Nigerians. In the 1970s, a Christian revival swept the country. ThankGod spent some time as a young man doing missionary work during this revival. He tells stories from this time of money appearing in pockets miraculously, just when it was needed. He and Julie knew each other slightly in Nigeria. They came to the U. S. in the late 1970s. Julie got a job working at a hotel. One day, armed robbers staged a hostage takeover at the hotel and shot several of the hotel employees, including Julie, whom they left for dead. She was not expected to live. Somehow she survived. She was not expected to walk again. Today the only remaining physical sign of this experience is a limp.

ThankGod visited her when she was recovering in the hospital. They fell in love. They also went to graduate school at the University of Massachusetts in Amherst, where they were married. ThankGod then went to work for a nearby state mental hospital. The couple started a small Bible study. It gradually became a small church. After holding services in rented hotel rooms and homes for several years, they reached an arrangement with the Northampton Grange to use their building as a church on Sundays.

The Grange is a fraternal agricultural organization which was once much larger than it is today. There are not as many farmers in Massachusetts as there used to be. The Northampton Grange owned a small old church building in Northampton, across the Connecticut River from Amherst. The Grange does not meet on Sundays. So they agreed to rent their building to Resurrection Life International Ministries for Sunday services.

We attended the Madukas' church for the last six years that we lived in Massachusetts. They kept in touch with us and prayed over the phone with us during Pam's illness.

The Madukas live in a large old house near the center of a small town near Northampton. One reason they bought the house was that the lot has enough room to build a church building on when they have enough building funds. We parked on the street and went around to the spacious back yard. Church members had rented an open canopy tent and a number of picnic tables. I was sure roast goat was on the bill of fare. The Nigerian community in western Massachusetts is large enough to support one or two goat ranches.

The pastors (Julie is as much a part of their ministry as ThankGod is) were dressed for the occasion. She wore a white silk top with a matching jacket, and he wore a simple white shirt and khakis. I saw some people who had left the church earlier under strained circumstances, who had returned for this celebration. Several of Julie's relatives in the States flew or drove to the party. At one point several of the relatives rose to sing some Nigerian songs.

They were dressed in the type of outfits you would see on the streets of Lagos. One man had on a light-blue gown shaped like a Protestant minister's robe. Another wore a tan-and-yellow shirt with bold African X's and triangles. The soloist was a woman dressed in a patterned pink wrap-around gown tied with a broad belt of similar material. Her hair was covered with a type of headdress we got used to seeing at church. It looked like the woman wrapped about a yard of material loosely around her head. Pam tried to do it once. She was not very successful. It is harder than it looks.

The songs involved a lot of rhythmic handclapping and nodding of heads. The crowd applauded at the end of each song.

A little later, the couple of honor reaffirmed their vows to each other. For his part, ThankGod got up to read a poem that he wrote himself. It was about six stanzas long. It praised God and Julie, in that order. ThankGod read the poem in a way that said he was serious but full of joy. No one giggled or tittered. I wiped my eyes at one point.

When they were free, the pastors came over and hugged us. A long time ago, I was uncomfortable when a man offered to hug me. Or a woman not my wife, for that matter. But it is the custom at Resurrection Life. There is nothing sexual about it, the way they do it. It is a natural thing to do. If a man hugs his sister with sexual thoughts in mind, there is probably something wrong with him. It is the same thing here.

Chapter 17

Chemo Begins

Pam was scheduled to begin chemotherapy the Monday after we returned from New England. A couple of weeks earlier, she had passed something called a MUGA scan, which had to do with checking the condition of her heart. Adriamycin, one of the chemotherapy chemicals, can damage the heart. If a person's heart is weak already, the oncologist does not want to be the one to push it over the edge. Pam's heart appeared to be rugged enough to take chemotherapy.

On that day, we drove up to Austin together and I dropped her off at her office. Then I drove on up to the Pickle Research Campus. I do not research pickles. The Pickle Research Campus is a University of Texas research facility named after U. S. Representative J. J. Pickle, who was instrumental in procuring funding for it. I worked on research for a few hours. Then I returned to Pam's workplace, picked her up, and drove to the cancer center for her appointment at a quarter after one.

The chemo room was just the way we remembered it from our visit. I watched as the Scottish nurse connected Pam to an IV, got some saline solution going, and then went off to get the first chemo drug. It was a clear fluid in a plastic bag. The nurse connected it to a tube going into Pam's arm. It took perhaps half an hour for the bag to empty. At the end, Pam felt fine. I thought that maybe this wasn't going to be so bad after all.

A feature I did not notice on our first visit to the chemo room was a fume hood in one corner. I am familiar with fume hoods— large cabinets with glass fronts and a strong exhaust that sucks out air from the top—from freshman chemistry class. If you are messing with something that is too toxic to breathe, you mess with it under a fume hood. I noted that the nurse was preparing the next syringe of chemicals under the fume hood while she wore rubber gloves.

She came out with a container that looked to my eyes like it contained about a quart of transmission fluid–reddish translucent stuff. It was Adriamycin. All that syringe was going in my wife's body. I told myself that they knew what they were doing. The nurse handed Pam a cup that held chunks of ice. She told Pam to suck on a piece of ice the whole time she was taking the Adriamycin. She said it would help to prevent mouth sores. I watched Pam as the Scottish nurse slowly injected the Adriamycin over a period of about thirty minutes. Pam read a mystery novel, sucked on ice, and acted like nothing special was happening.

Unless anything goes wrong, watching someone take chemotherapy is only slightly more interesting than watching paint dry. That time, nothing went wrong. Finally, Pam ran out of chemicals to take. The nurse unhooked her from the rig and gave her a prescription for some nausea medications. I hoped she didn't need them. We stopped on the way home at the pharmacy and got them anyway.

Suppertime arrived. Pam's appetite was normal. She ate lightly, not because she wasn't hungry, but because they told her to. It was a long day, so we undressed and went to bed early to read.

About 8 P. M., Pam sat up abruptly. She lost her cookies in the trashcan by the bed. It was over almost before I knew what she was doing. I asked her if she felt better now. She said she didn't feel that bad. All of a sudden she just had to vomit.

She had already taken one of the anti-nausea medications just a little while earlier. After she vomited, of course, most of it ended up in the trashcan. I carried the can to the bathroom, washed it out, and returned it to its place next to the bed. Around nine that night, we turned out the lights and went to sleep.

Around eleven, I woke up to hear Pam losing her cookies again. I held her head for a little while. She said she felt better. She took some more anti-nausea medication. We went to sleep.

At one o'clock, same thing. It took me longer to go to sleep that time.

At three, guess what. I asked her if there is anything I can do. She felt pretty bad that time. There was nothing to upchuck any more, but that did not stop her stomach from trying. I tried to get back to sleep.

In the morning she took two of the cheap kind of anti-nausea pills, and one of the expensive kind. This was the way they described them to us at the cancer center. I looked at the label of the expensive kind. It is called Anzemet. It cost somebody seven hundred and sixty dollars for ten pills. Our copayment was only forty dollars.

We were fortunate to have two incomes from organizations that provide some of the best health insurance available. I wondered what would happen if there were fewer people like us and more people with either no insurance or less generous insurance. Maybe Anzemet wouldn't cost seventy-six dollars a pill. On the other hand, maybe there would not be any such thing as Anzemet.

Pam took the Anzemet. It made her sleepy. It also reduced the nausea.

Tuesday morning, I did what I have done six out of the seven days of every week for my breakfast since about 1977: I put two pieces of toast in the toaster oven. Pam has never objected to this before. But when she came into the kitchen that morning, she said, "What did you do, burn up a cow in the stove? It smells terrible in here."

The chemo affected her sense of smell. She couldn't stand to be near anything with a noticeable aroma. She tried to eat and lost her breakfast. She didn't eat much the rest of the day. She drank some water and other fluids. The nurses told us it was important for her to drink several glasses of water a day after each chemo treatment.

By Wednesday, she was weak and dizzy. She didn't feel like eating. But if she doesn't eat, she will not get stronger. I called the cancer center. They told me to bring her in for a saline infusion. That took most of the day, with waiting, infusing, paperwork, and driving back and forth.

Before the infusion, they sent us in to talk to someone who appears to be in the line of social work for the cancer center. She listened while Pam told her what happened since the chemotherapy treatment. The first thing the woman said was "It's not supposed to be this way." Well, but it was.

She told Pam to drink plenty of fluids. I explained to her that Pam knew she should do this. But the anti-nausea medicine made her so sleepy that she was not awake enough to drink lots of fluids. And if she lays off the anti-nausea medicine, she is more wakeful, but she gets pukey again. The lady said that it's hard sometimes, but we should try.

We drove back home. Pam started to take more Compazine, the cheap anti-nausea drug. She wasn't nauseated as a result, but she slept most of the next couple of days. When you are sleeping, it is both difficult and inadvisable to eat. She felt a little better over the weekend. We looked forward to Monday, when perhaps she could go back to work. She was hoping before the chemo that at the worst, she would be a little tired for a couple of days after each treatment, maybe stay home a day or two, and then go right back to work. After all, that is what the typical experience is supposed to be. Instead, she was out a full week after this first chemo treatment. When she returned to work Monday, many of her coworkers assumed since it was summertime that she had just taken a vacation—perhaps to some exotic place like Acapulco, where she showed off her shorter, younger-looking hairdo.

Chapter 18

Downhill

On the following Monday, Pam did not feel like she could drive herself to work. So I drove her up to Austin and went on to the research lab. After work, she had an appointment at the cancer center to have a blood test. The official name for the test is a "CBC," which stands for complete blood count. These days, it is a while-you-wait process. Pam went into a side room off the main waiting area and chatted with a very pleasant phlebotomist, a woman from South Carolina. The woman took a little tube of Pam's blood with her down the hall and did something with it we never saw. A machine somewhere in the office analyzed the blood and printed out a page that Pam got a pink copy of. I could understand a few of the items on the page: things like "Name," "Date," "Physician." The other things were not obvious to the uninformed reader. There were a couple of graphs with wavy lines in the upper left corner and a square thing that looked like what happens when you fire a couple of rounds of buckshot into a piece of plywood: a scattered bunch of little dots. There were columns of abbreviations: WBC, NE%, LY%, RBC . . . . Down at the bottom, for convenient reference, there was a listing of the normal ranges for each of these numbers.

The nurse who handed this to us circled a few of the numbers. Pam's hemoglobin, white blood count, and neutrophils were all low. The nurse was most concerned about the neutrophils, which fight infection. Anything above 1.5 is OK. Pam's had gone down to 0.7. The nurse gave Pam a shot of something to bring her neutrophils back up. She said to come by Wednesday to have her blood tested again.

Wednesday the neutrophils were down to 0.3. The nurse said to come by both Thursday and Friday for more shots, and to get another blood test Friday—also, to stay away from crowds. Pam didn't feel like hanging around crowds much at that point anyway.

Friday, after two more shots, we anxiously awaited the latest pink sheet of mystery numbers. The nurse who brought us the results did not look pleased. The neutrophils went all the way down to zero. This did not look like progress. The nurse said for Pam to avoid crowds and mosquitoes. The West Nile virus was in the news. It is spread by mosquitoes. The cancer center was closed on weekends. The nurse told Pam to go to the hospital across the street, where they had a room for giving this kind of shot on Saturday and Sunday. So we came back to Austin Saturday.

The wisdom of telling patients whose immune systems are impaired to go to a hospital for a shot escaped me. But when we found the room, which was directly across from the elevator on the hospital's third floor, the nurse in charge told us that they used to have the booster-shot patients come into the general waiting room where all kinds of patients were hanging out. It finally dawned on someone that you didn't want infection-susceptible people mixing with infected people. So the hospital established this separate room for "neutropenics" like Pam. I was learning new words all the time.

The injection itself didn't take much time. But the nurse had to take Pam's temperature and observe her for a few minutes in case she had an adverse reaction.

The booster shots were called Neupogen. It is a type of hormone that stimulates the bone marrow to make neutrophils and other good things. It is a fairly new drug that was not available when my mother was taking an early form of chemotherapy in the 1970s, after the cancer came back for the second time. She just had to walk around shorn of her neutrophils.

Sunday, Pam's back started to hurt. By Monday her hips were

hurting too. The nurse said that this could be a side effect of the bone-marrow stimulation. I thought that maybe it meant something good was happening.

Pam felt too bad to go to work Monday morning, and didn't leave for work till noon. She stopped at the cancer center on her way up Monday afternoon to have her blood checked again. The neutrophils were now up to 14. According to the chart, the normal range was 1.4 to 8.3. Fourteen was better than zero, I figured.

About ten days after the first chemotherapy treatment, Pam began to lose her hair. At first it was barely noticeable. She did not wear her wig at night. In the morning there were some strands of hair on the pillow. Each time she washed her hair, it was noticeably thinner than before, especially in front and around the temples. But you see a lot of sixty-year-old women with hair that thin going around in public.

At the time, Pam was attending a prayer group at work that met every Tuesday at noon. The week of the neutrophil adventure, a man at the prayer group prophesied that Pam would not lose her hair. She did not remember him prophesying anything else before.

That weekend, we drove out to a small resort on the shores of Lake Buchanan. Our room was one of four in a cabin next to the parking lot. The room was furnished sparsely: an air conditioner, a bed, a chest of drawers, and some old photographs on the wall. One photograph showed a group of young people dressed in a way that dated the picture somewhere between about 1900 and 1915. The women had on long light-colored dresses and the men wore dark pants and white shirts. Some of the men wore jackets and a few had on hats. Several of the men without hats had slicked down their hair and parted it in the middle. They stood in a line outside a building that looked like a schoolhouse or perhaps a general store, with a long covered porch across the front. "Stood" is not the right word. "Danced" is better. They were lined up in couples, the women leading and facing right, the men holding the women's hands high. Several of the men's legs were bent or raised as if caught in the act of cakewalking. Everyone seemed to be having a good time.

When Pam combed her hair that evening, whole handfuls of it

fell out. She gathered it up and put it in the trashcan. We agreed that it was time for her to start wearing Samantha in public.

The cabins were on the edge of a rocky proclivity that led down to the shore where there is a gift shop next to a boat dock. Later that afternoon, we walked down a steep pathway through some woods and emerged into a clearing behind the gift shop.

The gift shop featured a long covered porch that faces the shore. There was a porch swing suspended by chains. We sat in the swing and watched the sunset. A boat buzzed by out in the middle of the lake. Like most manmade lakes in Texas, Lake Buchanan is long and relatively narrow. It is less than a mile wide at this point. We could see the woods and a few houses and docks on the other shore. It was peaceful. There were no doctors, nurses, IV machines, or waiting rooms. That is why we came.

Chapter 19

Six Thousand Dollars

On the following Wednesday, three weeks had elapsed since Pam's first chemotherapy treatment. It was time for the second one. She was still not used to wearing Samantha. The days were warm and the wig felt hot in the sun. The anti-nausea drugs slowed down her intestines, which made her constipated. The constipation gave her hemorrhoids, which she had never had problems with before. But after she didn't need the anti-nausea drugs–say the first week–she was able to get back nearly to what she remembered as normal.

At the cancer center, we checked in, waited most of an hour, and then were called to the chemo room. The treatment went fine. During the whole time she was undergoing chemotherapy, Pam never noticed any ill effects from the chemicals themselves at the time she received them. Some of the pre-treatment drugs bothered her in various ways, but not the chemo drugs.

She started taking the Compazine anti-nausea pills (the cheap ones) right after the second treatment. (She had held back some the first time, thinking she might not need them much.) They put her to sleep early Wednesday, but not so fast asleep that she couldn't wake up to vomit, twice.

Thursday she felt better, but was so sleepy from the Compazine that she barely ate or drank anything. I knew this wasn't good. But she looked so rested, lying there on the couch in the living room, that I hated to wake her up every hour to make her drink a glass of water. Even if I did, she usually wouldn't finish it. Before all this, when she was healthy she usually drank only three or four glasses of liquid each day, usually tea. She would make a glass of tea or soda at supper last till just before bedtime. So it was hard to get her to keep drinking fluids.

On Friday, we drove up to Austin to have the usual blood test. The nurse took a look at Pam and said she looked pretty puny. Had I been giving her enough to drink? I explained the problem. The nurse decided to give her an IV of saline solution to rehydrate her. While she was hooking Pam up to the machinery, she told me to make sure that she drank eight glasses of water a day.

"By the way," the nurse said, "your Blue Cross hasn't approved the Neulasta yet." Neulasta was an improved version of a neutrophil booster. The neutrophils were the anti-infection blood component whose number had drifted down to zero and then zoomed up to 14. Neulasta did the same thing as the daily injection, only you didn't need as many shots.

The nurse continued, "If you'll sign this waiver, we'll give it to her now, but if the insurance company won't pay, you'll have to pay for it."

"How much is it?" I asked.

"Six thousand dollars."

"For one shot?"

"Yes."

I could hardly believe my ears. The only other time in my life I felt the way I felt then was when I was talking to an accountant one February about my income taxes. He misunderstood something I said and told me that I owed twenty thousand dollars in back taxes. I did not have twenty thousand dollars at the time. It took a few minutes to clear up the misunderstanding. They were long minutes.

I asked the nurse what the alternative to Neulasta was. "Well, the Neulasta will do her until the next chemo. With the Neupogen you have to have a shot every day for five days." Neupogen was what had made Pam's back and hips ache.

I asked Pam if she could stand to come back every day for five days rather than run an unknown risk of having to pay six thousand dollars. She said yes, she could stand it. In the meantime, the cancer center would wait to hear if Blue Cross would pay for the six-thousand-dollar shot.

That was on a Friday. That evening, Pam had some mashed potatoes and jello. She said that for a change, they didn't smell like burning rubber or chlorine. (Some foods did smell that bad to her for several days after a treatment.) Then in the middle of the jello, it all came back. She said she had swallowed the wrong way. I didn't think that was the real reason, but I didn't disagree with her.

That evening, I drove to a nearby hardware store to get some filters for the air conditioner. The huge store covered most of a city block. I looked for the particular size I needed but didn't find it.

After some searching, I saw an employee of the store talking to a customer in an aisle. The employee was a young woman a little shorter than me, stocky, and wearing a bandanna on her head. She was talking to the customer about chemo treatments. I waited until the customer walked away. I asked the young woman where to find the filter size I needed. She showed me. Then I asked her if she was undergoing chemotherapy.

She was—for breast cancer. She had been in treatment since May. She had five of her six treatments. She said she occasionally got a little queasy. But she had never missed a day of work.

I once read about a theory of human personality that was based upon body type. The three types were the ectomorph, the mesomorph, and the endomorph. The ectomorph type was thin and tall. The mesomorph type was muscular. The endomorph type was stocky and short. Pam tends toward the ectomorph category. The young woman in the hardware store was definitely an endomorph. Maybe that was why she wasn't bothered that much by chemo. Or maybe not.

Chapter 20

Breathless

A week or so later, Pam began to have a new problem. For the last several years, my university has held a picnic on or about Lyndon B. Johnson's birthday, which is August 27. LBJ is the most famous graduate of the school. There is a wide gap between him and the next most famous graduate, whoever that might be. The picnic is held on the spacious lawn of the university president's house. On the day of the picnic, Pam said she was feeling well enough to go. The closest parking space I could find was down a steep hill a couple of blocks away. Pam had to stop and get her breath a couple of times on the way up and down the hill.

It reminded me of my father during the last year of his life. He showed very few symptoms of the lung cancer that was to kill him. But he gradually got short of breath more and more often. The only complaint he voiced was, "I feel like if I could just get my breath back I'd be okay."

Pam had a chest X-ray as part of her preparation for chemotherapy. It showed nothing unusual. But her shortness of breath frightened me. It went away once she got in the car and rested a while.

The week after the picnic, the fall semester began. The day after Labor Day, Pam went to the cancer center to have her blood tested.

A red blood cell count that was supposed to be at least 10 was down to 9.3. This caused the nurse to give Pam a shot of Procrit, which was supposed to boost her red blood cell count.

The Wednesday of the second week of September was September 11, a year after the attack on the World Trade Center. That day, I had a lab I needed to supervise at the university until noon. That morning, Pam told me that she would be fine taking the chemo on her own this time. So she drove up to Austin, worked half a day, and then showed up for chemo at two that afternoon. Much later, she told me what had happened that day in more detail.

First, she saw Dr. Smith, who asked her how she was doing. He did this before every chemo treatment.

She was not feeling that well this time. Her rear-end problem (hemorrhoids) were getting worse, she was getting a sore throat and a cough, and her energy level had not come back to normal. She asked him what her blood count numbers were this time. He looked through some papers and told her. They were lower than they had been before her previous treatment.

She asked him, in light of the lower numbers, whether she was eligible to take the next chemo treatment.

He replied, "Oh, you're always eligible to take chemo." So they went ahead with Chemo Number Three. She went back to work afterwards. Then she drove home, ate supper, and lost her cookies again.

This time, the nurses had sent her home with a third combination of anti-nausea drugs to take: something called Kytril, another one called Torecan, and for emergencies, some Phenergan suppositories. The nurses said to give her Phenergan only if she couldn't keep down any of the oral pills, because it would knock her out for several hours, guaranteed.

Well, that evening, she vomited at six, at seven, and at eight. I asked her if she wanted a suppository. It would be a painful process to take one, but she reluctantly agreed. In the last week or so, her difficulties in that area had become so painful that I heard her scream once or twice in the bathroom. When I asked her what was wrong, she said that she was just going to the bathroom and it hurt like hell. The suppository hurt too. It put her to sleep in about fifteen minutes.

The next morning when I woke up, she was still lying in exactly the same position that she fell asleep in. Previously, she had told her boss she wouldn't be in for the rest of the week. I let her sleep and tried to work at home.

The previous Sunday, we had visited my sister in Fort Worth. On the way home, we stopped in Hillsboro where there is a big outlet mall. Pam said if she had a kitchen timer, it would help her drink a glass of water every hour like the nurse was recommending after chemo. We found a little electronic one in a kitchen accessory store and bought it. So after she woke up around nine that Thursday morning after the third chemo, I set the timer next to her on the couch where she was lying. She set it every hour and drank the glasses of water I handed her.

As for food, she felt too bad to eat anything solid. At the drugstore I found something called Boost-Plus, which is a liquid nutrition drink for invalids. She managed to drink one of those for lunch and another for supper. The new anti-nausea drugs did not make her quite as sleepy as the other ones. I thought things were going fairly well.

I had to teach a lab that evening. When I got back about half past eight, Pam was already asleep.

Back when we lived in Austin during my graduate-student days in the early 1980s, I would often ride my bicycle the four miles or so between our duplex and the campus. Ever since then I had longed to live close enough to my job to ride a bicycle. When we moved to San Marcos, we found that the town itself was so small, it was hard to find a house that was *not* within biking distance of the campus. So I bought another bicycle and began riding it to work once or twice a week.

The next day, a Friday, Pam seemed to be doing well enough for me to ride my bicycle to campus to teach a lab. The early fall weather was still quite warm. The ride took about twenty minutes.

After the lab, I was in my office typing on my computer. The phone rang. It was Pam. She wanted me to come home. She felt really weak and was having trouble breathing. I told her I'd be home as fast as I could. I wish that I had noted the time I left campus on my bike and the time I got home, because I am pretty sure I set a record that day which I will never surpass.

She was lying on the couch in the living room. She looked very pale. Her lips were slightly bluish. Sitting up cost her an effort that made her breathe hard. When she went to the bathroom she had to hold onto the walls to steady herself.

I called the cancer center. Pam was already scheduled for a blood test that afternoon. The nurse said if Pam was well enough to get into the car, that I should just take her up there at the regular time. The trip takes the better part of an hour. She said if Pam was really bad off to call an ambulance and take her to the South Austin hospital. I hung up and wondered what "really bad off" amounted to.

I told Pam what the nurse told me. She said she would try to get dressed to go. She managed to get down the hall into the bedroom. Then she collapsed flat onto the bed, breathing hard. In broken sentences, she said she just couldn't do it.

If she couldn't get into a car, and she was doing this badly, I didn't know what else to do but call 911. So I did.

The emergency medical services van arrived in about ten minutes. By then Pam had made it down the hall and onto the couch again. Two young men came in through the open front door. They hooked her up to a portable monitoring machine. They peered at it for a few minutes and said her heart looked good. Then they loaded her onto a fold-down gurney, rolled her out the door, and said for me to follow them. They seemed pretty happy that she wasn't any worse off than she was.

They didn't turn on their lights or run their siren. In fact, they took a pretty leisurely route to the hospital. Pam later told me that they started her on an IV and some oxygen in the ambulance. I pulled up behind them and followed them inside.

I was able to stay with her in the emergency room the whole time. Most of it was spent in a curtained-off cubicle next to a man who was having his bleeding stomach pumped. He appeared to be in the last stages of alcoholism. You never know who you will end up next to in an ER. If your own problem is not imminently fatal, there is usually someone there worse off than yourself.

From time to time, various medical staff people came by. The first was a registration person who wanted Pam's Blue Cross card and a lot of information. The next was another nurse who took her vital signs and a vial of blood. Next came the ER physician, who asked her a few questions and found out who her oncologist was.

We could hear voices as far as several cubicles away. At one point we heard Dr. Smith's voice. He was telling someone a joke about a leprechaun on a golf course. But he never stopped by our cubicle, then or later.

In about an hour, the ER doctor came to take Pam for a couple of lung tests Dr. Smith had ordered, including a scan in which she breathed xenon gas and a chest X-ray. Her lungs looked normal. Her blood test was confused by the IV and the extra oxygen she had breathed on the way to the hospital. The ER doctor said he wasn't sure what was wrong. But she was feeling better now. He let us go about suppertime. We were glad to get out of there. Pam had a Boost-Plus and I cooked myself something that did not smell strongly. Then we went to bed.

Pam went to sleep at once. I lay awake thinking. The fact that the chest X-ray was clear told me that the cancer had not spread to her lungs. Or if it had, we couldn't see it. At any rate, her breathing problems were not due to cancer. They were due to cancer treatment. I wondered how much more of this Pam can take.

When I cannot sleep, sometimes I recite the 23rd Psalm silently. It is not magic. But it is something to do. When one is saying mentally that the Lord is my shepherd, I shall not want, it is difficult simultaneously to worry in a coherent way as well. Eventually I went to sleep too.

Chapter 21

Dammit, Do Something

During the days after our trip to the ER, Pam did not improve much. Her stomach was unsettled enough to make her vomit once a day over the weekend. She was able to eat some solid food after that. She got on the scale and found that she had lost fifteen pounds since the chemotherapy began. And she was not fat to begin with.

By Wednesday of the following week, seven days after the third treatment, her mouth and throat were so sore that it was uncomfortable just to breathe. I took Pam to the cancer center to be looked at. After the usual blood tests, we were sent in to see their nurse practitioner, the one I thought of as the staff social worker.

The impression I received from this woman was that she had to handle a great many patients every day. To deal with them, she had boiled down her job to a set of stock phrases: "chug-a-lug that water" and so on.

Pam described her symptoms. The woman did not seem to take them that seriously. She just repeated the same phrases about drinking plenty of fluids and eating right. She seemed surprised that Pam was having any problems. Pam's throat was so painful that drinking water was becoming a challenge. Although the woman had Pam's chart in front of her, Pam had to point out to her that she had lost fifteen pounds since the start of therapy.

The woman said she would prescribe something called "triple mix" which should take care of the throat pain. When we stopped at the facility's pharmacy on the way out, they said there wasn't anything for Pam. It was not clear to me what to do after that, since all the people in authority were off on other appointed business. It would probably mean another forty-five-minute wait to get the problem straightened out. We had to get back to San Marcos. So we just left without the triple mix.

That night, Pam tried propping herself up on pillows so she could breathe more easily and with less throat pain. It helped some. Thursday night she woke up shortly before midnight. She could not get back to sleep. She moved onto the couch in the living room so that I could sleep.

The next day, Friday, I had to go to work to run another lab. Pam was in constant pain from the soreness in her throat and her rear-end problem. She was starting to have trouble breathing again. So before I left for work, I decided to set up another appointment at the cancer center to see what they could do for her.

The cancer center was a busy place. But I supposed that they were equipped to deal with emergencies such as this one. I called their main number and told them we couldn't get there until the afternoon because I had other obligations. The woman on the other end told me there were no openings that day. At all.

I lost my temper.

I said, "Dammit, you've got to do something."

The woman said, "Hold on a minute, Mr. Stephan, let me finish. We may be able to do something but I'll call you back."

"All right. But hurry up, please."

In about five minutes she called back. The only thing she could offer me that day was a time slot in their Round Rock office. Round Rock is about fifty miles away, north of Austin. We knew nobody in the Round Rock office. If we had been going to Round Rock all along, I suppose we would have taken this as a matter of course. But we hadn't been, and we didn't.

When I held the phone and told Pam what they were saying, she said it would be easier to get in to see her general practitioner, Dr. Mallett, who is closer by, in South Austin. So I told the cancer center to forget it, we'd call her GP. And I did.

When they heard what the circumstance was, they said the doctor wasn't in that day, but his nurse practitioner could see Pam at a quarter after eleven. That was in the middle of my lab, but I told them fine, we'd be there. I went up to the lab at the scheduled time of 10 A. M. I got everyone started and told them they were on the honor system and to turn in their lab reports under my door when they were finished. I had to take my wife to the doctor. They understood.

I returned home and put Pam in the car. We drove to the GP's office. The nurse practitioner's name there was Lisa. She listened to Pam and looked at her throat. When it was time to examine the other end I excused myself. As I stood in the hall, I heard Pam say, "OW!" once. After a suitable interval, I knocked and they let me back in.

Lisa prescribed some powerful ointment for the back end and triple mix for Pam's throat. On the way out of the office to our car, Pam stopped to vomit. There are some times when the only thing to do is watch. I stood by until she said she felt like traveling. Then we got in the car and went by the pharmacy on the way home. The triple mix turned out to be a milky pink substance that numbed everything it touched. It did help Pam's throat. She slept better that night.

Saturday and Sunday, Pam's shortness of breath continued. She felt too bad to go to church, so I stayed home with her. We had a minor obligation there that day, so I called the pastor's wife Nancy to tell her we wouldn't be coming so she could make other arrangements. A few minutes later, Father Len called back to ask if we would want him to come down to give us communion after church. I said that would be good.

Pam had not been able to keep any food down for the last two days. It is not an easy thing to sit in the kitchen eating a sandwich for lunch when your sick wife is a few feet away on the couch, unable to eat anything. Around two that afternoon, the doorbell rang. It was Father Len and Nancy.

He was dressed in his black suit and reversed collar, and carried a small communion kit. He set it up on the coffee table beside the couch. Pam was glad to see them. She sat up long enough to participate in the abbreviated service. After that was done, Nancy suggested that we pray for Pam. So we stood around her and prayed for her problems and for healing. I thanked them for coming and they left.

About four that afternoon, Pam said she felt feverish. I took her temperature. It was 101.5. The cancer center had a standing rule that if a patient ever had a temperature over 101 to call them right away. This time, I was following their own rules.

I called their number. An answering service took my number. In a few minutes a doctor I didn't know called back and listened to my description of the situation. He wanted to prescribe a broad-spectrum antibiotic. By this time it was about six in the evening. He asked me to give him the number of a San Marcos pharmacy that was open. I said I would find one and call him back. I called around and discovered that there was no pharmacy open after six on Sunday evening in San Marcos. When I called him back with this information, he said to bring her in tomorrow.

That evening and Monday morning, she tried to eat something. It all came back—four times. She was clearly deteriorating. Using Pam's high temperature as a lever, I was able to pry open an appointment at the cancer center for half past one that afternoon. I left her at home while I went to work to give my Monday lecture. I returned at noon and helped her into the car. The thirty-foot walk from the couch to the garage exhausted her.

The wait at the cancer center was only a few minutes, for a change. When they called her name, I helped Pam stand up and held her arm as we went past the nurses' station. She was bent over and very pale. Dr. Smith was in the area when we came in. I saw his face change expression when he caught sight of Pam. I told him I wanted to talk with him later in the week. He scurried off down the hall.

A nurse took a blood sample and started Pam on a saline IV. It did a little good. She was still having trouble breathing. In a few moments, here came the same nurse practitioner we had seen the week before. She addressed Pam, who was lying there with an IV in her arm, and started to talk about forcing fluids again.

I got mad. At a break in the conversation I leaned forward, looked the woman in the eye, and said, "Look, we're doing the best we can. But you folks have tried this and that and she's still getting worse all the time."

What I said was probably not as significant as the way I said it. The woman lost her fixed smile and said, "Wait a minute, I'm sensing some hostility here. I'm only trying to help. Part of the problem is that Pam hasn't been telling me all these problems earlier when they came up first. You need to communicate better. Don't hold back anything. If patients didn't complain, we'd have nothing to do and we'd lose our jobs!"

After a few more tense words, the woman moved Pam from the examining room where they had hooked her up to the IV to the chemo room. She was still on the IV. They told us that they were waiting for some test results. We waited.

A couple of hours later, the Scottish nurse showed up with some papers in her hand. She gently told us that Pam's hemoglobin count was 7. The minimum standard for normal life was 15. This meant she should go straight across the street to the hospital and check in to get a blood transfusion. The papers were the orders for this to happen.

At the hospital, they told us they were full at the moment. But something might open up later in the day. It was about four in the afternoon. It was beginning to look like we were in for an all-night procedure, and we had not so much as a toothbrush with us. So I gave the admissions desk person our home phone number and asked them to call us when an opening showed up. Then we drove home.

I ate another solitary meal. Pam concentrated on breathing. We hoped and prayed for the hospital to call. Out of curiosity, I called the local San Marcos hospital and asked if there was room. They said unless our doctor was associated with them, they couldn't help us. So there.

Around eight that evening, the phone rang. There was a room available. We put a bag in the car and drove back up to Austin.

The process of receiving a transfusion is more complicated than it used to be. We took the order with us—a stack of papers with the words "thrombocytopenia" and "anemia" prominently displayed at the top. That was what was wrong with Pam. They took the papers away. This initiated an elaborate process that was described to us by the male nurse who administered the transfusion about two o'clock the next morning.

First they typed Pam's blood and crosschecked it with the transfusion blood. Then two different people had to sign off on the process, checking her wrist tag with the bags of blood. Then she had to sign another pile of papers by which she acknowledged that she understood all the possible adverse consequences of this blood transfusion, up to and including death. Then, and only then, he started the transfusion.

Late-night conversations are different than normal conversations. As the night nurse watched one pint after another disappear into Pam, he told us how he got to like the night shift when he was doing aeronautical meteorology in the Air Force. The weather does not sleep, and so someone has to keep track of it even at night. He became accustomed to working the night shift. After getting his nursing degree, he transferred his preference in shifts to medical work. He liked the feeling of independence and quiet that the night shift gave him. When he finished with the last bag and packed up his equipment, we were almost sorry to see him go. I settled down on a kind of folding bed the room featured and tried to go back to sleep.

The next day, Pam felt much better. She felt well enough to think about what would happen next. We talked about it.

After the first two treatments, she had briefly considered calling a halt to the whole process. But then she got better and decided to continue. She felt better now. But she still did not want to have more chemotherapy. We did not look forward to telling Dr. Smith this. He stopped by quickly the next morning just long enough to tell Pam that he thought she should stay until Wednesday.

Later that day when he came by again, he sat down on the arm of a chair across from Pam's bed. He clearly wanted to talk. We let him.

He was apologetic. He said when the program started, there was no intention of landing Pam in the hospital. He admitted he wasn't sure why Pam was not doing better than she was. But he was now considering more options, including "deep-sixing this whole chemo business." I was glad to hear that he was thinking about it too. He said Pam's reactions were in the one-percent category of very fragile constitutions that could not take the standard six-treatment regimen. He said he would stop by again the next day. If she was feeling better, he would let us go home.

That afternoon, I drove down to San Marcos to teach an evening class. Pam's friend Tammy Martin asked her mother Sharon to stay with Pam for that time. So between Sharon and me, Pam always had some company during her whole hospital stay. I returned about nine that night, Sharon went home, and I spent the night in the hospital room with Pam.

When Dr. Smith came by Wednesday, he said to set up an appointment with him for the following week to discuss the next step, whatever it might be. Then he signed Pam's release papers. We went home.

The following Saturday, there was another shape-note sing, this time at an auditorium in San Marcos. Pam said she wanted to go. I took her there. The atmosphere was quite different in a modern auditorium than it was in a century-old church. Halfway through the program, Pam asked me to take her home. She was feeling too tired to stay.

When we got home, she started to cry. She said she didn't know if she would ever get better. She wanted to get better, but her throat still hurt, her butt hurt, and she could hardly walk without getting out of breath. I mostly listened. In the past, I have tried to argue her out of things that made her feel bad. This rarely works for men. It almost always fails for women. Just listening is harder sometimes, but it works better.

Chapter 22

Retreat

Pam stayed home the entire week after that. As soon as the treatments began, she had applied for something called a sick leave pool at her job. People who are healthy donate their extra sick leave hours to the sick leave pool. Some staff people in charge of that matter then decide who receives the surplus hours, based upon need. Pam's condition was life-threatening if not treated, so that took priority over people with less serious conditions. We heard around this time that she had been granted 720 hours of sick leave. Pam had used a considerable amount of this during September because she had been sick so much. Her boss told her that she needed a doctor's note saying it was okay for her to go back to work when she was ready to return. We had a choice of doctors, so we decided to ask Dr. Smith. We also wanted to talk with him about what to do next besides the same kind of chemotherapy she had been having.

I phoned the cancer center. I began to notice a pattern. The receptionist could connect me to a therapy nurse, or to their prescription office, but whenever she connected me to the appointment staff person, that person never answered the phone. Instead, I heard a recording saying that I should leave a message and that they would call back. I always left a message. But they didn't always call back.

Pam and I made two or three tries to get some action out of them over several days. I considered getting in the car and driving up there, but I had other things to do such as teach classes. And Pam didn't feel like driving herself yet.

On Thursday a week after the transfusions, one of the nurses at the cancer center called and asked Pam why she hadn't shown up for her ten-thirty appointment. Pam said that nobody had told her she had any ten-thirty appointment. The nurse said, "Wasn't that your voice on the answering machine?" We never received the phone message on our answering machine. The nurse must have called the wrong number and left the message on some stranger's machine. It would have been funny if it hadn't been so annoying. Pam asked to speak with the appointment nurse to set up another appointment. She got connected to a recording.

By Saturday, Pam was ready to get outside the house. I proposed that we drive down to San Antonio and visit the Oblate Renewal Center, a Catholic institution that includes a seminary and some other organizations. I had been there several times but Pam had never seen it. She agreed. We drove the hour or so it takes to get to the north side of San Antonio.

I found out about the Oblate Renewal Center from a Catholic friend who I talked with when I was looking for a good place to make a private retreat. With my training in mathematics, the first thing I thought of when I heard the word "oblate" was a spheroid flattened at the poles. The same Latin word also means "worshipper" or "one who makes a sacrifice."

The Oblate Renewal Center is on a large plot of land in a residential area of San Antonio. You drive up a one-way street that leads to a Catholic school and seminary and turn into the center's parking lot. The architecture is modern mission-Hispanic: stucco walls, arches, and lots of sunlight, at least when the sun is out.

My favorite place in the Center is the grassy area behind the main building, between it and the seminary. There are some large old trees there and a path that winds between some rustic plaster sculptures that are Stations of the Cross. Stations of the Cross aren't my thing. But this is one of the few park-like places within many miles where a person can sit and read a Bible, close his eyes and think or pray, and even cry, and no one will bother you. I have done all of these things there at various times.

Pam was with me that day, so I just played the tour guide. I showed her the Lourdes grotto. According to a brochure you can get at the Center, it is an exact reproduction of the place in France where the Virgin Mary appeared to St. Bernadette. There are statues of these two parties posed in the appropriate positions, and a large rack of candles nearby. Behind the grotto is a chapel where they expose the Host for veneration, but I didn't go in. Pam did.

We left after about an hour or so. Pam was feeling well enough that day to cook supper. I was grateful for two reasons: (1) that she felt well enough to cook and (2) that I didn't have to eat my own cooking again. I had been doing all of the cooking whenever Pam didn't feel like it, which was most of September. Both Pam and I survived my cooking. But it is not an experience I want to repeat.

Chapter 23

Dr. Kilbourn

The Monday after that, Pam called the cancer center to make sure she had an appointment to see Dr. Smith. They told her that not only did she have an appointment to see him, but they had made another appointment in the morning for her to come get her blood tested and her chest X-rayed. If she hadn't phoned early, she would have missed the earlier one altogether. She drove up to the cancer center and went on to work for a while. I drove up to meet her in the lobby after lunch in order to see Dr. Smith with her. She was still determined to say she didn't want any more chemotherapy.

The doctor showed up with a sheaf of papers in his hands–the results of the blood test and chest X-ray Pam had taken earlier in the day. We asked him what the options were at this point. He held up his hand and said, "Wait, wait, wait," and kept looking through the papers. Now and then he mentioned this or that result. Finally he looked up and said, "Okay. Options."

One option was to skip any more chemotherapy altogether, and go on to a long-term cancer-preventing drug such as tamoxifen. That was a possibility, but he said he would feel like he wouldn't be "giving you your money's worth." A better choice, he said, would be to go to a milder type of chemotherapy called taxol, which he would administer once a week for three months.

He said we didn't have to decide right away, and to set up another appointment in about a month. If we wanted to start with taxol, we could start as soon as a week from then. We had planned a weekend trip out of state for a week later, and so we said we'd want to take that trip first. He said fine. After our trip we'd talk with him again.

Some time earlier, Pam had learned about a group of women with breast cancer who got together once a month or so and just shared experiences. She began to attend their meetings as she was able to. After our talk with Dr. Smith, Pam called a few of her friends from the breast cancer support group and told them the story of the last few weeks. One woman had never heard of anyone landing in the hospital like that from chemo. Another woman said that Pam ought to get a second opinion about the advisability of further chemo. We had gotten tired of having to drive forty miles to Austin and back every time a doctor wanted to see her. So Pam looked in her Blue Cross preferred-provider book to see if there were any oncologists in San Marcos. There were. She called the office of a Dr. Kilbourn. The receptionist was happy to set up an appointment for her to see the doctor the following Monday afternoon, when I could go with her again. So when Monday came, we drove the ten minutes or so from our house to Dr. Kilbourn's office.

The Southwest Regional Cancer Center is in a small building at the edge of the divide between East Texas and the Hill Country. To the east the land is mainly flat, grassy plain. To the west you can see the buildings of downtown San Marcos and the university against a backdrop of tree-covered hills.

We went inside. There was no one else in the waiting room. The receptionist (one of two) greeted us pleasantly and settled the copayment. Then she said a nurse would be with us in a moment. Already, I liked the SWRCC better than the other cancer center.

After the preliminary checks of height, weight, and so on, we met Dr. Kilbourn. He was our age, late 40s or a little older. He wore a tweed jacket and a serious but not unkind expression. His manner was quiet and respectful to the point of diffidence. He listened as Pam described the course of her treatment up to that time. From time to time he made sympathetic noises. When she got to the point where she had the fever the Sunday evening after Father Len's visit, he said he thought that they should have sent her to the hospital then, not a day later.

He agreed with Dr. Smith that continuing chemotherapy with the less astringent Taxol would be a good idea. But unlike Dr. Smith, he gave us a reason. Chemotherapy is not simply a blind assault on all of a person's systems in the hope that some cancer cells will be killed in the process. The treatments are timed to attack the generations of cancer cells at the most vulnerable point in their life cycle. When the process is successful, the number of cells is reduced by a certain factor after each treatment, and the law of geometric decrease goes into effect. For example, suppose 90% of the existing cancer cells are killed during each treatment, if timed properly. And suppose they divide once between each treatment, doubling in number. After six treatments, the number of cancer cells is reduced by a factor of (0.1×2) to the sixth power, which is 0.000064. But if you wait too long between treatments, the cells get a chance to multiply more than once and the advantage goes away. Dr. Kilbourn's point was that if Pam stopped now, she would not get much if any benefit from the chemotherapy that had been done so far. It would all be a waste.

When Dr. Kilbourn expressed the situation in that way, it put the matter in a different light. We went home and talked. When I reminded Pam what the nurse practitioner at the old cancer center said about patients needing to complain so the staff could keep their jobs, something snapped in her. She said she could not go back there. She was going to transfer to Dr. Kilbourn. I was glad.

We wrote a letter to Dr. Smith which thanked him for his services thus far. We said we had found a doctor closer to our home, and that we were transferring to the San Marcos doctor.

Chapter 24

The Hair Returns

On Monday, October 28, we went to meet with Dr. Kilbourn again. There was one other person in the waiting room. We waited about five minutes. When he came into the examining room, Pam told him that she wanted to go with the low-dose Taxol, which was one of the options he had mentioned at our last meeting. He said fine, that we could start as soon as next week. She asked to start on a Wednesday, so she could have at least two days a week at work even if she was wiped out over the weekend. Dr. Kilbourn explained that he would give her the chemotherapy once a week for three weeks, and then give her a one-week rest. He said that this way the body gets to recuperate more than if he went all the way through without a break. In his experience, he said, patients usually ended up with the need for suspending the treatment somewhere along the line anyway. If he planned for it and built it into the schedule, he said things usually went more smoothly. It sounded good to us.

One side effect of taxol is temporary damage to the nerves that can result in tingling and numbness in the extremities. He said glutamine, a harmless food-quality amino acid, seems to alleviate these symptoms. He asked us to buy some glutamine and for Pam to take three teaspoons a day during the day of chemo treatment and for three days immediately afterward. We could get it at a health-food store. In San Marcos later that the week, I bought a pound of glutamine for forty-four dollars. At three teaspoons a day, it would last for quite a while.

The next Wednesday, I drove from the university to the SWRCC office and met Pam for her first taxol treatment. After checking in, we met Lea, the chemotherapy nurse for the day. She turned out to be an eight-year breast cancer survivor. She spent nearly her entire afternoon tending to Pam. Once she got the IV inserted, she told us about how hard it was for her to be a chemo patient after being on the other end of the needle for years. But she thinks the experience made her a better nurse.

The chemo room at SWRCC was on the corner of their building too. But instead of looking out on a parking lot and the backs of some neighboring business buildings, the view from the rear window showed a wide-open field: tall grass and sky.

Lea explained that sometimes people have an allergic reaction to taxol. In order to prevent it, she was going to administer some Benadryl through the IV first, along with some Anzemet (an anti-nausea drug) and some other things. Lea said the Benadryl was likely to make Pam sleepy. It did. She got so dopey she could barely talk. But then she got anxious that she hadn't taken her teaspoon of glutamine yet. She had brought some with her in her bag, so I got it out and mixed it and gave it to her.

That calmed her down for a bit. Then she began to shake all over. She said she felt like she was freezing. Lea put a blanket over her and waited. She said it was probably a mild reaction to the Benadryl. Pam got anxious about what was happening. The doctor on duty (not Dr. Kilbourn) asked me if I thought Pam should have a tranquilizer. I took him out in the hall and explained that she generally wanted to get by on the fewest drugs that would do the job, and to wait a while. He did. Pam got better. In about an hour after inserting the IV, Lea began the Taxol.

Pam had no trouble with it. She went home and ate normally that evening. There was no nausea and no vomiting. If anything, she was more energetic than usual for a day or so afterwards. Lea had mentioned that one of the drugs was a corticosteroid, and might have this effect. The Anzemet made her constipated. That aggravated her rear-end problems. But overall, the Taxol was a great improvement over FAC. Saturday she began to feel rather tired. After church on Sunday she took a nap most of the afternoon. But that was the extent of the effects that we noticed.

The next treatment went even better. Lea didn't give Pam as much Benadryl as she did the first time. Pam didn't develop the shakes. She had no nausea. Her appetite improved. She began to try to gain back some of the weight she had lost. Like most women, she had maintained for years that she was about five pounds overweight. But she had lost that plus ten more by this point. So she wanted to get back at least to what she considered her ideal weight.

By the week after that, Pam was feeling so good about the new treatment that she told me I didn't have to come to the third one. But I showed up anyway. Lea wasn't there this time. The new nurse didn't look at Pam's blood test results before she hooked Pam up to the pre-medication IV. Pam asked what the test results were. The nurse looked at them. Then she said, "Uh-oh, your neutrophils are too low for you to have chemo today. I'm going to give you a Neupogen shot instead. I won't charge you for the pre-meds." So it was back to daily Neupogen shots for the next four days. The six-thousand-dollar Neulasta shots would not work with the low-dose weekly Taxol cycle, so that issue never arose.

A week later, Pam's neutrophils were up enough for her to continue with Taxol. A strange thing began to happen with her hair.

It had begun to fall out about ten days after the first FAC chemotherapy treatment, back in August. It continued to get thinner and thinner for the next several weeks. By the time Pam went into the hospital for the blood transfusions in October, she was nearly bald.

Around that time she began to wear a kind of nightcap with an elastic band when she went to bed. Her eyebrows and pubic hair also disappeared. The only hair that endured all chemical assaults was the hair on her forearms. But she wasn't fond of that hair anyway.

As I write this, I am trying to recall an image of how she looked without hair. It is difficult. Some women with a lot of nerve and a desire to look constantly as if they were walking down a runway at a high-fashion show can carry off being bald without a problem. It fits what they want the world to think their personality is. But Pam is not that way. She wore Samantha, her nice wig, in public, a cheaper but more comfortable wig around the house, and the nightcap to bed.

Once or twice, she showed me what her head looked like without hair. It was bald, all right, with just a trace of fuzz and a few straggles of short hair near the back.

One night shortly after she commenced Taxol, she turned to me in bed and said she wanted to show me something. I got interested. She took off her nightcap and said, "See? It's coming back." Over most of her scalp there were little bristles. It reminded me of the way my father used to have me cut his hair. He was about half bald, and did not want to spend much time tending the other half. So every few weeks he would get me to put a kitchen chair out in the garage. He sat down in it and I got out some electric clippers and gave him a burr. It was a lot like mowing the lawn. What was left was about an eighth of an inch long and stiffer than bristles on a toothbrush.

Pam's hair looked and felt a lot like that. The sensation of lying next to my father's skull in bed was not a pleasant one. I told her I was glad her hair was coming back, but could she please put her cap back on. She understood.

Chapter 25

Thanksgiving

Thanksgiving was coming. Back when we lived in Massachusetts, we could never convince anyone from Texas to join us for that holiday. So we did not have a Thanksgiving with family, other than each other, for the whole time we lived in Massachusetts.

Once we moved to Texas, we began to share Thanksgiving with my sister's family. We decided to hold it in alternate years at her house in Fort Worth and at ours in San Marcos. One reason for this was that her two children could be with her for Thanksgiving only every other year. Her first husband divorced her in 1994. He lives in Fort Worth and their son Matt lives mainly with him. At the time, Laura, the daughter, lived mainly with my sister, whose name is Liz. After her divorce, Liz married a male nurse named Mike, who was as different from her first husband as it is possible to be in many ways. They are happy together. We had reason to be happy with them on that Thanksgiving.

On the long drive up to Fort Worth, I had time to think. I thought about other holidays.

There was the last Christmas my mother was alive, in 1979. She spent it in the hospital. I remember it mainly from pictures we took at the time. In the pictures she is propped up in the hospital bed, smiling, with her wig and glasses on.

There was the last Christmas her only sibling Judy was with us, in 1991. Judy had been diagnosed with lung cancer and had undergone chemotherapy that had removed her long lustrous black hair. But a year or two earlier, she had come down with a flu that had the unexpected side effect of making her quit drinking. (She had been an alcoholic for decades.) The change in her personality was astonishing. Judy's mother (my grandmother) summed it up at the time when she said, "I have Judy back again." The Christmas after she was diagnosed, we visited her during our short annual holiday trip to Texas. She sat on a chair in her den with a stylish scarf on her head and said she was ready to live or to die, either way. But she was content and at peace with herself and with God. A month later, she was dead.

My sister is a nurse by training. She began her nursing career in the emergency room of a large municipal hospital. After a few months in such an environment, she got to where she could keep going with something close to a good attitude in almost any circumstance. Perhaps she always had that ability and the emergency room just brought it to the surface. Except for a few occasions during her divorce, I have found her in a positive, energetic state of mind no matter what was happening. She came down to visit us once during Pam's illness and helped us negotiate the unfamiliar decisions involved in Pam's treatments.

Laura was fifteen that year. She was a beautiful, slender, blonde young woman with dark brown eyes. This is not just family prejudice talking. During the Thanksgiving meal, Liz told us how on a lark, she and Laura answered a cattle call for teenage models in Dallas. Out of some 400 girls they photographed and briefly interviewed, the agent in charge invited some 50 to come back. Laura was one. She and her mother were discussing the next step, which would be to fly out to the agency's headquarters in Hollywood for more pictures.

Matt, who was twelve, was unimpressed by these doings. He had not quite gotten to adolescence yet. He had been living mostly with his father for the last six months after a bitter custody battle in court that my sister lost the previous spring. Fortunately, when we saw Matt that evening at Thanksgiving dinner, we saw that Liz's worst fears about her ex-husband's influence on Matt had not come to pass. Recently, Matt had begun to send me emails that he mass-mails to everyone on his email list. They were usually little inspirational stories that concluded with an exhortation to email the story to your best friends. I didn't mail the emails to anyone. But I was glad he emailed them to me. He never asked me what I did with the stories.

After the meal, Matt retired to his room to play a computer game. Mike turned on the TV, which was playing "Indiana Jones and the Temple of Doom." It is the darkest and least enjoyable of the Indiana Jones films. But I watched it out of lack of anything else to do. Laura and Pam disappeared into Laura's room. Laura had a big project for English class which consisted of a series of interviews with someone she admires. She has chosen to interview Pam.

The day after Thanksgiving, we drove over to see my Aunt Percy, who was living for the time being with her daughter Marcy in Marcy's condo. During the previous six months, Percy went through a clinical depression and received electroshock therapy, which brought her out of it. A side effect of electroshock therapy is temporary short term memory loss. With Percy looking on and smiling, Marcy told us the story of the day she picked up Percy from the hospital after the electroshock treatments. Percy got in the car hopping mad that her husband Perry wasn't picking her up instead. There was a good reason for this, of course, which was that Perry had died two years earlier.

It took Marcy some time to work up to explaining how things were to her mother. But Percy took it pretty well. Marcy laughed, patted her mother's leg, and said, "Yep, our little nut case." Percy described her plans for later in the year to meet the same group of women she has met with one way or another nearly every year since they all graduated from Ole Miss (Mississippi State) in 1947.

The next week, Pam resumed her Taxol treatments. For the last month or so, her left shoulder had been acting up. She realized that she was unable to move it in certain directions. The one-week chemo respite gave her time to see a specialist about the problem. It turned out to be something called a frozen shoulder.

The doctor explained it this way. The shoulder joint is rather like a ball-and-socket joint held together by a shell of sinews and tendons. (Those are not the technical words for them, but that is what they are.) These tendons look like the strands of a rope. When the arm moves in different directions, the tendons twist like a rope being twisted to allow the motion.

In the case of a frozen shoulder, scar tissue and inflammation around the joint bind some of the tendons together. They can no longer slide past each other freely. The result is that the shoulder's motion becomes limited. We looked up the subject on the web. No one knows exactly why frozen shoulders occur. But inactivity and illness can contribute to them. Pam had both.

There are different things that can be done for frozen shoulders. Physical therapy can help. Sometimes a surgeon can go in and cut the tendons free. Or sometimes a therapist takes an anesthetized patient, grabs the arm, and simply forces the joint to move beyond its limits. This last treatment is no longer so popular as it once was, because occasionally it breaks the arm. And sometimes the condition goes away on its own after a year or two.

Pam decided that she has had enough surgery for the time being. She chose to go to physical therapy once a week. Her therapist periodically measured the three directions of motion with some special instruments. After several visits, the therapist reported slow but steady progress.

During Pam's Taxol treatment the week after Thanksgiving, Dr. Kilbourn told her to go get five Neupogen shots before her white cell count started to fall. That way she would be less likely to get into serious trouble. We were glad to do it.

On Saturday, December 7, we drove up to Austin for Pam's Neupogen shot. On the way back, we stopped at the San Marcos Evening Lions Club Christmas-tree lot to buy a tree. San Marcos is a relatively small town, much smaller than Austin. But it has more than its share of fraternal organizations such as Lions Clubs, Odd Fellows, and Kiwanis clubs. There are two Lions Clubs: the Morning Lions and the Evening Lions. I imagine the Morning Lions as frisky, energetic go-getters, and the Evening Lions as sedate, contemplative, and laid back. The Evening Lions we meet at the Christmas tree lot are good old boys wearing checked shirts and canvas gloves. Their trees are all labeled by type and height with color-coded labels.

We picked out a tree that is about my height and reasonably symmetrical. Since we plan to put it against a wall in the house, it was okay if it had a good side and a not-so-good side. Pam agreed with my choice. I wrote a check to the San Marcos Evening Lions and loaded the tree into the back of my pickup truck. Pam stood by and watched, since her frozen shoulder and general physical condition were not up to helping me carry a tree.

During Pam's chemotherapy, I gradually took over various jobs that she used to do: cleaning out the catbox, washing, drying, and sorting the laundry (including her things), collecting and carrying out the trash, and (until recently) cooking. Cooking was the first thing I was glad to give back to her. But I still kept doing the other things until Pam asked to do them again.

We drove home and I wrestled the tree out of the truck. I went up in the attic and carried the box of Christmas decorations down the narrow folding stairs that drop down into the middle of the garage. I found the four-legged Christmas tree stand, the good one, not the old three-legged one that we have nevertheless not thrown away yet. As I screwed the screws into the trunk of the tree, I told Pam, "You know, when they were going through General George Custer's effects after he died, they found one of these."

"Really, a Christmas tree stand?"

"Yup, you know what it was?"

"No, what?" I could scarcely believe I had brought her this far.

"Custer's last stand."

She picked up a hammer and pretended to go after me with it. This told me that she was really feeling better. A month earlier, she would not have smiled. And a month earlier, I did not feel like telling her jokes.

Chapter 26

Markers

During the next two months, life kept approaching what we remembered as normal. On a week when Pam received Taxol on Wednesday, she would get tired by the weekend and take a nap on Saturday or Sunday. Her rear end continued to give her problems, and her frozen shoulder did not improve much despite the physical therapy. But she felt well enough to plan and give a Christmas party for some of our university friends, to travel to Fort Worth to be with my sister's family for Christmas, and to get away for a couple of days to a state park built around a power-plant reservoir. Her job provided about a week of automatic vacation between Christmas and New Year's. This allowed her to rest when she felt like it.

The Taxol treatments were scheduled to end in February. Toward the end of January, Dr. Kilbourn added to the usual blood tests a tumor marker test. Tumor markers are proteins that are associated with the presence of certain types of cancers. The association is a loose one. This means that people without cancer can sometimes show high tumor marker numbers, and people with cancer can show low tumor marker numbers. But he felt it was a good thing to do. At the time we thought nothing of it.

On Thursday, January 30, I was working in the lab in Austin when the phone rang. It was Pam.

She said, "Are you sitting down?"

I sat down. "What's the matter, are you all right?"

"Dr. Kilbourn's office called and left a message for me to come in and see the doctor tomorrow, and be sure and bring my husband."

She was upset. I got upset. I dropped what I was doing, left without locking the lab door behind me, and rushed down to her office on campus. Two of her friends from a prayer group were there with her. She had been crying. She was too upset to call the SWRCC people back to see what the matter was. So I did.

I got Lea, the nurse who had first given Pam the Taxol. Lea explained that one of the tests for tumor markers they had done the day before had come back unexpectedly high. She had asked Dr. Kilbourn if this was a "scramble." He said no. I told her that when we heard the phone message, we immediately expected the worst. "Don't get ahead of us here," she said. Dr. Kilbourn would explain it to us tomorrow.

Pam was too worked up to do anything more at her job that day, so I took her home. We spent an hour looking up tumor markers on the Web. We found out that they do not always mean cancer. But they can be an indication of it. This information helped us calm down enough to sleep that night. But we were eager to hear Dr. Kilbourn's words the next day, and we could barely wait to see him.

When he came into the examining room that day, his face betrayed no concern. He explained that the test he had run was for something called CA-27.29. Around Oct. 8, someone (presumably Dr. Smith) had ordered a test for this marker. Normal was between 20 and 30. Pam's had come out about 52. That is high, but not that unusual for someone who has had cancer and is starting chemotherapy. Dr. Kilbourn had just run the same test and had gotten back a number that was almost exactly the same: 52.9. So what did it mean?

He said it bothered him, because if the marker really indicated cancer and the chemo was getting rid of the cancer, why wasn't the number going down? Occasionally, he said, a person's liver would become impaired by chemotherapy and this would cause the tumor marker number to be high. And other things besides cancer can make it read abnormally.

The only thing he would change, he said, would be to move up the CT scan and the bone scan he was planning from three months to six weeks from then. These tests were to check for any signs of cancer after the end of the chemotherapy treatment. Also, if there was no problem, they would serve as reference scans that later scans could be compared with. We thought that was a good idea. We went home feeling better.

Pam was still wearing her wig to work. It had fooled most of the people most of the time so far. Her hair was now longer than a burr, but shorter than the shortest haircut she would like to be seen in public with. It was also long enough to show a much darker color than her former medium blonde shade. But, as she put it, hair is hair. She was glad to be getting any back at all.

One afternoon, a young woman came by Pam's office and asked her where she got her hair done, because it looked so nice. Pam could tell this was not what the woman really wanted to know. So she told her the whole story, cancer and chemo and all. The conversation led from cancer, to longevity, to the woman's grandmother, who lived to be ninety-nine. By that time, the grandmother was living in a rest home. She was mentally fine and spent much of her time reading. One day she was reading a book with her door open. Her room was directly across the hall from a nurse's station. Suddenly she looked up and straight out the door, apparently at a nurse who happened to be standing there.

The grandmother said, "Nurse, there's a man with piercing eyes standing in my doorway. Would you ask him to go away?" Then her head dropped down on her chest and she died.

Back when we were not sure that death wasn't imminent, Pam would not have wanted to hear a story like that. But I was encouraged that she could at least talk about it again without losing her composure.

Chapter 27

Sex And Other Things

By the time of Pam's last Taxol treatment, she was feeling better than she had felt in a long time. Unlike the FAC, the Taxol treatments did not make her feel worse and worse. The one-week breaks between the three week sessions of chemotherapy seemed to help in this. The Friday after her last treatment was Valentine's Day. We had supper by candlelight at home, with shrimp and asparagus she cooked herself.

If you are a man, you may want to know about what happens to the sexual aspect of a relationship when the woman has cancer treatments. Clinically, Pam was nearing, or perhaps in, menopause (lack of menstrual periods) when she was diagnosed. The chemotherapy treatments had the side effect of sending her into menopause, which is not uncommon. That, plus the Tamoxifen she began to take after the chemotherapy was over to prevent recurrence, gave her mild to severe menopausal symptoms such as hot flashes, vaginal dryness, and other problems.

We managed to deal with these problems. I can tell you attitudes I could have had which would not have helped. Some men demand sex as a right without thinking of the woman's needs, desires, physical condition, or state of mind. In my experience, this attitude always causes trouble sooner or later, usually sooner. Other men react to a situation like Pam's by shutting off altogether sexually, refraining even from touching her for fear of hurting scars or causing discomfort, or simply out of a gut-level feeling that can almost amount to revulsion. If the resulting abstinence is too great to bear, they find alternative outlets such as pornography or another relationship. This approach is just as bad as the first one. It tells the woman she is no longer loved.

Shortly after Pam completed chemotherapy, I read an article in a magazine about a woman who had advanced breast cancer. When she was dealing with a recurrence of the cancer and was feeling her worst physically, her male partner told her that he was leaving. After telling her physician this bad news, she said, "I always knew he was weak." That is not the way to go either.

My task was to show Pam my love in ways that were appropriate to the situation. When she felt good, that could include sex. When she did not, it could still include kisses and hugs. You can kiss a woman even if she is lying in a hospital bed, or at least hold her hand and tell her you love her. That is the message she will remember.

When Pam felt bad physically, there was another thing we could do in bed together: watch movies and eat popcorn. Every week or so we rented a movie and watched it together. When Pam was ill at home, she would sometimes watch a movie by herself. But whenever I was home we would watch one together.

I tried to suit the movie to the occasion. When she was feeling emotionally down, I looked for silly comedies. One night we watched a Laurel and Hardy film called "The Devil's Brother," made in 1933. It was full of physical stunts. One of the major comic roles was played by a bull. It got her to laugh. Another film we watched together was the original "Odd Couple" with Walter Matthau and Jack Lemmon. It was one of the two or three funniest movies I have ever seen. Watching a movie tired us out, especially if it ended late at night. So we didn't watch more than one or so a week. But it was something to look forward to on weeks filled with chemo and Neupogen shot appointments.

Another thing we did together was cooking. On the last Tuesday of February, it began to sleet. By eight o'clock that morning it was only 26 degrees outside, and we heard on the radio that both Pam's university and mine were closed for the day. So we stayed inside and baked cookies for a party we held the following Saturday for a new professor in my department.

The next week, Pam came down with a cold. Even though she had finished with her chemotherapy treatments in February, her white blood cell counts were not back to normal. We called Dr. Kilbourn and he prescribed an antibiotic for her to take. It did not have any adverse consequences and kept Pam's cold from getting worse. But not before she gave it to me.

Around the middle of March, Pam went to have her CT scan and bone scan to check for any signs of cancer. I was teaching and couldn't go with her. The procedures were not difficult. They told her that they would give the results to Dr. Kilbourn in about a week. At the same time, they took a blood sample to test for the tumor marker that had been 52 before. We prayed that things would come out good.

Thursday, March 20, marked a year since the day that Pam had the mammogram that told us she probably had cancer. I drove Pam to work and went on to my research in Austin. When we came home, the blinking green light on our answering machine told us we had a phone message. I went down the hall to put up my things while Pam stayed in the living room to hear the message. In a moment I heard Pam yell something. I rushed back down the hall. She was smiling and jumping up and down like she had won the lottery.

"Listen to this! Listen to this!" She played the message again. It was Dr. Kilbourn. He had received the test results from the scans and blood tests. He said the results were "excellent." He gave no further details. But we trusted him enough to know that if he said the results were excellent, the details wouldn't matter that much.

On the following Monday, we went to see Dr. Kilbourn to hear the details anyway. The CA-27.29 tumor marker number was 28, which was entirely normal. And nothing suspicious showed up on her bone and CT scans. He could not explain the earlier high numbers for the tumor marker except to say they were "lab results."

On the way home from the doctor's, I remembered something that happened the day Pam had the tests that gave the good results.

I spend about twenty minutes every morning praying. Usually Pam is still asleep then. The morning of the tests, I was praying as usual, and prayed that Pam's test results would be good. I received a strong impression that I should get up, go into the bedroom, and lay my hands on Pam and pray for healing so she would have good results on the tests. There was no voice, no odd sensations, just a definite idea. I went ahead and did it. Pam woke up briefly and thanked me when I explained what I was doing. I will never know what might have happened if I had not obeyed the impression. But I am glad I did.

Chapter 28

Easter

After Pam was diagnosed with cancer, we started to hear about all sorts of people in the same situation. First, there was the breast cancer support group that Pam met with many times. They gave her the sense that she was not alone in the situation, and helped her decide to change oncologists when the time came. Next, there were people we knew who felt free to tell us of their past experiences with cancer once Pam told them about her situation. There was an old friend of mine in Massachusetts who was a fellow engineering professor. It turned out that his mother had died of breast cancer when he was a teenager. His sister Joanne was diagnosed with breast cancer a year before Pam was. When he heard about Pam, he put her in touch with Joanne. They exchanged mutually encouraging emails. And then there was Geneva, who had been diagnosed with stomach cancer just before Pam had her mammogram.

After Geneva was released from the hospital, her Austin oncologist told her that she needed aggressive chemotherapy, which would make her quite ill. To get a second opinion, she went to the M. D. Anderson Cancer Center in Houston. The doctor there advised her that in order to preserve the quality of whatever life she had left, he would recommend a certain milder type of chemotherapy in pill form. He also estimated she might have two or three months left. She followed his advice. She resigned all her volunteer positions at church. Later in the year, she and Walter joined their son and his family on a Caribbean cruise.

She knew about Pam's situation. Whenever we saw her at church, she never failed to ask Pam how she was doing with her chemo. About a year after her diagnosis, Walter told us that Geneva was not taking the chemo any more because it had done all the good it was going to do. All Geneva would tell us about herself was that she felt tired a lot and took long naps in the daytime.

Easter came late in 2003, on April 13. Father Len preached on the resuscitation of Lazarus. He contrasted it with the resurrection of Jesus. Jesus rose on his own; Lazarus needed help. Jesus never died again after his resurrection; Lazarus presumably died some time or other after his resuscitation. The point was: would you rather be resuscitated like Lazarus, or resurrected like Jesus?

We usually sit near the back of the sanctuary. That day I looked around at the crowd, which was larger than usual. I saw lots of people I didn't know. There was a young man sitting next to a woman we knew. The woman had asked us the week before to pray for her son. He was living with a young woman who had turned him against his mother. The mother was worried that she might never hear from her son again. Not only did the son show up at church that day, but beside him was a woman who looked like she was his girlfriend. Something good had happened there.

Toward the front, there were two men in wheelchairs. One had been coming for a while. At first I didn't recognize the other one. Then I realized it was Joe.

Joe used to come regularly when we began attending the church about three years earlier. Then we heard he had contracted spinal cancer. He never showed up any more, but his wife and children kept coming. I remembered Joe as a relatively tall balding man with a slightly hooked nose. The man in the wheelchair had the same bald head and hooked nose. But the rest of him had withered and twisted. At the end of the service, he stood up with some help. He was about six inches shorter than the last time I had seen him. His head tilted and his upper body had a semi-collapsed look to it. He smiled and shook hands with people right and left as his wife followed him a few steps behind with the wheelchair. Something was here that he really wanted to meet. It was in the people, but it wasn't just the people. I was glad to see him.

The Robert Benton film "Places in the Heart" begins with a shooting, continues with a lynching, and winds up with a tornado. In between the viewer is treated to a raw image of small-town Texas as it was in the 1930s. It was the Texas my parents grew up in.

The last scene in the movie takes place in a church during the serving of the Eucharist. Everyone is singing a hymn. The camera first shows some ordinary people dressed in their shabby Sunday best. Then we see some musicians who seem a little out of place: they are dressed in their flashy performing clothes. Finally, we see the black boy who was lynched at the beginning of the film. He is right there, alive and well, singing along with the rest of them.

We are not told in detail what Heaven will be like. The pictures of harps and golden streets probably express in analogical language things that human speech is incapable of dealing with directly. But I think Robert Benton's picture is a good one. Easter Sunday 2003 at St. Francis Episcopal was another good earthly image of the kingdom of Heaven.

Geneva was too ill to come.

Chapter 29

Geneva's Good-Bye

By Easter, Pam was feeling well enough to do most of the things she had quit doing when she became ill. She began to fold her own laundry again. She began to clean out the cat box herself. I still carried out the trash. Her left shoulder was still frozen. This made it hard for her to reach high shelves and to put on certain clothes. So I helped her with these things. But in many other ways, she was recovering well.

The Sunday after Easter, we missed seeing Geneva again, and Walter her husband as well. On the last Sunday of the month, Father Len told us that Geneva was getting very weak. Experience told me that if we wanted to see her again, we had better do it soon. We called and Walter said Wednesday afternoon would be a good time. Pam made some split-pea soup and vegetable salad. I went up to Austin that afternoon and we drove to their house after Pam got off work.

Over the last year or two, Walter had told us something of their lives together. They had met and married when they were both teenagers living in a small town in East Texas. After the war, Walter became an accountant with an oil company in Houston. They raised two boys, one of whom died in an accident when he was in his twenties. The other son became an ophthalmologist and set up a practice in Austin. After Walter retired, he and Geneva moved to

Austin to be near their grandchildren. That was twelve years earlier.

Their house in North Austin was in a neighborhood of garden homes with small yards. The street in front was smaller than a regular city street, but wider than a driveway. Walter answered the door. He was dressed casually, not in the gray suit and tie we always saw him wearing at church. He invited us in to see Geneva. She was lying down in the bedroom.

The first thing I noticed in the room was a pair of large photo portraits. Each showed a young man of high-school age with long sideburns. They hung above the bed where Geneva lay with her leg propped up on some pillows. She was suffering from incipient phlebitis, Walter said. But from her tone of voice and facial expression, Geneva did not appear to be suffering at all.

We sat down and talked, or mostly listened, for half an hour or so. Shortly after we arrived, the doorbell rang again. It was a hospice staff person. Today was the day that the hospice people were going to start their services. There was a piece of oxygen machinery on the floor next to the bed. Geneva explained that they had just moved it in that day. Neither she nor Walter knew how to work it yet. Walter excused himself to talk with the woman from the hospice.

As soon as Walter left the room, Geneva began to tell us about several times that Walter had been seriously ill. Once he was misdiagnosed with an intestinal complaint. Another time he broke his ankle. The doctor put on the cast too tight. He developed phlebitis. It landed him in the hospital for seventeen days. That was back when she was working as the head accountant for a one-man oil production firm. At vestry meetings, Geneva always understood the treasurer's report quickly and could point out mistakes or inconsistencies. Pam had wondered where Geneva got her excellent head for accounting figures. Now we knew.

Walter returned in a moment. It was clear that he, Geneva, and the hospice woman wanted to talk for a while. We excused ourselves and went into the living room.

It was very neat. There was a large television and above it a reproduction of an oil painting. The painting showed Jesus as he rode a donkey into Jerusalem on the first Palm Sunday. Walter had explained how he and Geneva had asked their children and grandchildren not to buy them any more Christmas presents because "we don't have that much room here, and there's just not anything more we need." But he had relented when his son bought them the picture.

When Walter and the hospice woman came into the kitchen, he said we could go back and talk with Geneva some more. We stayed about five minutes longer. Then we noticed that she looked a little tired. Walter came back into the room. Pam asked if we could pray for Geneva. They said it would be fine. Pam prayed for healing and encouragement. Then we said good-bye.

On the way out, Walter told Pam that it was a fine prayer. It was the last day of April.

On Tuesday, May 13, Father Len emailed us that Geneva had had a stroke. Walter had gone in to wake her up and she had not responded to him, although she was still breathing. Two days later, we sat down to supper and the phone rang. At that time of day it is very likely that a telephone solicitor is on the other end. But I picked it up this time. It was Father Len. Geneva had died about two that afternoon.

Chapter 30

Why?

On the way to Geneva's funeral the following Monday, Pam hoped that it would turn out better than the Episcopal funeral of the father of a high-school friend of mine. Father John Hildebrand had been the parish priest at an old, established Episcopalian church in downtown Fort Worth for many years. He died the summer we moved to Texas in 2000. My sister read about it in the paper and called me. We drove up to Fort Worth for the funeral. I had not seen my friend for twenty years. The last time I heard from him was when they announced that they had had a baby boy.

That funeral was conducted strictly by the book. Depending on which psalms and prayers the priest in charge selects, the Book of Common Prayer's Order for the Burial of the Dead can be as short as five or six pages. The person in charge of Father Hildebrand's service chose most of the short selections. There was no eulogy or other personal mention of the deceased except for the times when his name had to be read according to the book. Outside the church afterward, I saw my friend, his wife, and a college-age young man next to him who had to be the baby. It was not a time to criticize funeral styles. We just hugged them and told them we were sorry.

Later, Pam objected to the depersonalized way that funeral had been run. I expected that this one might be a little different.

The body was nowhere to be seen, neither was there a casket. But the body was no longer the focus of attention. Father Len followed the prescribed text up to a point. Then he said that Geneva and Walter would have been married for sixty-two years next Thursday. "You don't do that on your own. It requires supernatural help–and that's what they had." He spoke of how she had given faithful and diligent service to the church, to the Altar Guild that she founded when the church began a dozen years earlier, and to him personally. He said that when she resigned her positions upon her diagnosis fourteen months ago, he felt like his right arm had been cut off.

But it was the right thing to do, he said. She spent the last year of her life living it. She enjoyed being with her family. She rarely if ever complained. It will sound strange to say this, he said, but she had a beautiful death. It was peaceful, without struggle, and showed that at all times she knew where she was going.

He had to stop at one point. Some people think a man who cries is weak. What I saw was a struggle for self-control. It is fitting to want to cry when someone you love has died. But it is also fitting to fulfill one's duty to one's parishioners. Duty won, but in a way that showed the love too.

Afterwards, a woman who knew Geneva well came up to me and said, "I like going to funerals where what they say is *true*! Haven't you been to funerals where you're not sure they're talking about the person you thought they were?"

On the drive home, I wondered why Pam was still here and Geneva was gone.

There was the statistical answer: Because old people are more likely to die than young people. But there are plenty of young people who die, and plenty of old people who manage to put it off for a long time: the ninety-nine-year-old grandma who finally saw the man with piercing eyes, for example.

There was the medical answer: Because they found Geneva's cancer when it was too late to do much about it, but they found Pam's when it was treatable. But there are some people who are diagnosed with Stage Four cancer and survive, and there are others who die of cancer that was treated when it was still in Stage One.

There was the religious answer: Because God allowed it. But why? Those who don't believe in God, don't believe that this is any kind of an answer at all. Those who do may still want to know an answer to the question, "Why?" Although we do not have an answer yet, we can hope that some day we will see God, for whom there is nothing unknown. But how he answers the question will be up to him.

Chapter 31

Lessons

When I finished writing the book up to this point, I handed it to Pam to read. After she finished, she asked me what I would have done differently if we had to do it all over again. I thought of several things.

First, I would have been more forceful about getting her to have a mammogram once her breast problem didn't go away. If she had had a mammogram as soon as she had some discomfort and felt a lump, it would have been smaller. She might have been able to get away with only a lumpectomy and radiation without chemo. This would have saved her hair as well as her life.

If that hadn't happened, I would have listened to my instincts more when we met Dr. Smith for the first time. I had a distinct negative reaction when I met him for the first time. I have had the same kind of feeling at certain other first meetings. In nearly every case, it has turned out that I haven't gotten along with the parties involved. It would have been much easier at that point to switch oncologists, or at least to get a second opinion.

And I would have arranged to be with Pam when she went for her mammogram that produced the bad news. It was hard on her to be alone then.

On the other hand, there are several things we experienced because of her condition that I am grateful for. It seems to be a rule in this life that nothing good comes without at least the possibility of pain or loss. Living as we do in a prosperous country where we are protected from most routine dangers, we can easily forget this truth until an unplanned and unwanted bad thing happens to us.

The film "Master and Commander" is based on Patrick O'Brian's historical novels about Captain Jack Aubrey, who commands a British man-o'-war in the early 1800s. It has inspired a movie critic (Anthony Lane of *The New Yorker*) to say the following: "What the novels [and the film] leave us with . . . is the growing realization that, although our existence is indisputably safer, softer, cleaner, and more dependable than the lives led by Captain Aubrey and his men, theirs were in some immeasurable way *better*–richer in possibility, and more regularly entrancing to the eye and spirit alike." Life back then was—on average—painful, exhausting, and short. But for those who survived, and perhaps even for those who did not, there was the reward of knowing that they suffered for a purpose: the glory of the Crown, the protection of their fellow seamen, or simply to do the right thing when it came time to do it, whatever the cost.

The first time I visited the Oblate Renewal Center, I met a nun whom I shall call Sister Hildegarde. She was in her late sixties, I suppose, with an Irish lilt to her voice and an enthusiastic manner. She invited me into her office for a few minutes. We chatted about who I was and what I wanted to do along the lines of a private retreat, which was entirely fine with her. Each time I returned after that, she would chat with me first for a few minutes and then I would go on about my business for the day. Eventually I realized that now I had a spiritual director, although that was not my original intention.

Once I figured this out, I felt free to tell her what was going on in my life, especially after Pam was diagnosed. Sister Hildegarde was sympathetic and encouraging in a way that I knew was sincere. In later visits, I found myself telling her that the cancer experience had brought Pam and me closer together. This did not surprise Sister Hildegarde. God is good at taking bad situations and turning them into good outcomes, she said, even if the basic situation doesn't change.

It may not be too much to say that the same principle applies to all of life. I have spent much of my life avoiding trouble: being a good student, not breaking rules, not driving too fast, getting a safe engineering degree that made me employable, fitting into organizations instead of rebelling, eating right, not wasting money, staying out of debt, and so on. I have made it to the age of 50 by living this way. But I have to admit that the times in my life that have made the most difference, both in the lives of others and in my own life, have been times when I took a chance or did a risky, even dubious thing, and stayed with it to discover the outcome. We once traveled to the Philippines during a time of political unrest when most Americans were staying away. The trip cemented a relationship with friends that has lasted until this day. I could have gone to a safe in-state college and no one would have objected except for a strange high-school English teacher I had who thought I could do better; I ended up taking her advice and going out to California to a school where I did not know a soul. I had a fairly secure engineering job four years later; I quit and went back to school to get my Ph. D. And so on.

Pam did not choose to get cancer. But once she had it, we had a risky, dangerous situation thrust upon us. I could have cut and run away. Some men do. It would have been cowardly. Except for certain subcultures such as the military, courage is a neglected virtue in today's padded, over-secure world. The challenge of Pam's cancer was a call for us both to exhibit courage. I could have done better, certainly, but I am grateful for the chance to have been there for Pam when she needed me.

Pam asked me what I would have done differently. I have asked myself what I am glad I did, and what things helped me get through the situation.

God. Faith is something God gives that we receive. Some people never have it. Some people have it early on, lose it, and never ask for it back. As a boy, I had a kind of cheap-plastic-import faith until I went to college and received the real thing. Which was good, because it was tested a few years later during my parents' illnesses and deaths. It was tested again a few years later during a difficult time in my life when faith seemed to be a problem more than an answer.

Like bones in a living body, faith that withstands stress becomes stronger. Because of the faith that was given me, I knew going into this thing that God would see us through somehow, and he did. Many people without faith manage to endure cancer of their own or in someone they love. But there is nowhere to turn in that case besides other people, and other people can let you down. Faith made a tremendous difference to me.

Regular habits. This sounds dull. But I mentioned before how the doing of routine little things like taking out the trash or washing the car can help you get through a difficult time. Faith has enabled me to maintain a daily cycle of meditation and prayer each morning. I have done this for so long that I cannot say what my days would be like without it. But as badly as some of my days go, I expect that the average would be much worse without meditation and prayer. When I was angry during Pam's diagnosis and treatment, I took this time to confess the anger to God and ask him for freedom from it, or for wisdom about what to do about the situation. When I was fearful, I took time to tell God about it and ask him to give me courage. And when we received good news, I thanked God in this time. Besides spiritual exercise, I take regular physical exercise, swimming or bicycle riding two or three times a week. I also fast from time to time. I like to think of fasting as a way to remind my body that I do not live by bread alone. Trying to keep these habits in place during Pam's illness gave me something to do besides sit and worry, and kept me in spiritual and physical shape to take care of her.

What happens next, I don't know. As of this writing, Pam is healthy, and I am healthy. I thank God for every day that Pam is free from cancer. But Joe, the man whose spine was crippled by cancer, died a week ago Monday. There are things we can do nothing about, but we can always choose how to act in the face of them. I know that whatever happens, there will be choices to make. Some of those choices are right and some are wrong. I hope and pray that we will have the courage to choose the right ones.

Chapter 32

Postscript

Of This Sad Time was written in 2004, a couple of years after the events described in the book. I am glad to report that as of now (October 2015), Pam is alive and well, and her hair is longer than it was in 2002 before chemo, though somewhat darker. It is still her most distinguishing physical characteristic. Her latest mammogram showed no sign of cancer, for which we praise God.

Not long after she completed her treatment, she quit her job at the University of Texas and eventually found employment with an online information service called About.com, editing their breast-cancer section. This was a way that she could put her experience with cancer to good use by helping others in a similar situation. It was a job she could do from home, which was fortunate, because in 2006 her father Ben moved in with us. His wife, Pam's mother, had died a year previously, and Pam's sister contacted us to help her deal with her father's progressive Alzheimer's disease. After looking at the situation, Pam decided the best thing would be for Ben to move in with us, and he did. Pam became his full-time caregiver.

The story of how that went might make another book, but not yet. Ben passed away in February 2015 at 89, and less than two months later, Pam's only sibling, her sister Phyllis, died at 52 of an aggressive bile-duct cancer.

Back in 1994, when we were still living in Massachusetts, Pam and I had the opportunity to work as volunteers at a restoration project in Oxford, England at The Kilns, for many years the home of C. S. Lewis. The organizers arranged tours of historic sites nearby, including Holy Trinity Church in Headington Quarry, where Lewis is buried. It's a small, peaceful churchyard shaded with trees that made it fairly cool even on the hot July day when we visited. The headstone is just a flat slab with a cross. Underneath the cross are these words, written by Lewis's brother Warren:

IN LOVING MEMORY OF

MY BROTHER

CLIVE STAPLES LEWIS

BORN BELFAST 29TH NOVEMBER 1898

DIED IN THIS PARISH

22ND NOVEMBER 1963

MEN MUST ENDURE THEIR GOING HENCE.

The last line is from *King Lear*. It is spoken by Edgar, the son of the Earl of Gloucester, as he leads his blinded father in a flight from enemies who will kill both him and Edgar if they don't flee. Gloucester—old, tired, and discouraged—has just said, "No farther, sir; a man may rot even here." Edgar, despite the dire circumstances, calls on his father to show courage, and shortly afterwards defeats his wicked brother Edmund in a swordfight.

In 2002, Pam and I didn't know if it was time for her to go hence or not. But we stood together, and with God's grace we endured her battle with cancer. Despite all the medical advances of the last thirteen years, people still get cancer, and some of them die of it. We can do what we can medically to fight it. But just as important as the medical battle is the kind of thing Edgar did for his father: to be there in time of need, and to encourage the sufferer. That is what I tried to do for Pam. That is what Pam did for the readers of her online breast-cancer site. And I hope reading this book has been an encouragement for you to do the same.

About The Author

Karl Stephan was born in Fort Worth, Texas, and educated at the California Institute of Technology (B. S.), Cornell University (M. Eng.) and the University of Texas at Austin (Ph. D.). He has taught at the University of Massachusetts Amherst and Texas State University, San Marcos, Texas. He has worked for MIT Lincoln Labs, Motorola Inc., and Scientific-Atlanta. His research areas have included microwave systems, atmospheric physics, plasmas, the history of technology, and engineering ethics. He has published over seventy papers and book chapters, and blogs on engineering ethics at http://engineeringethicsblog.blogspot.com.

Other books by Karl Stephan include:

Analog and Mixed-Signal Electronics

Karl D. Stephan

ISBN-13: 978-1118782668
ISBN-10: 1118782666
Edition: 1ˢᵗ, April 6, 2015
Hardcover Textbook, $105.88
Available also as a Wiley E-text and on Kindle
536 pages
Published by Wiley
Available on Amazon, Wiley, Apple iBooks, Google Play

A practical guide to analog and mixed-signal electronics, with an emphasis on design problems and applications.

This book provides an in-depth coverage of essential analog and mixed-signal topics such as power amplifiers, active filters, noise and dynamic range, analog-to-digital and digital-to-analog conversion techniques, phase-locked loops, and switching power supplies. Readers will learn the basics of linear systems, types of nonlinearities and their effects, op-amp circuits, the high-gain analog filter-amplifier, and signal generation. The author uses system design examples to motivate theoretical explanations and covers system-level topics not found in most textbooks.

Provides references for further study and problems at the end of each chapter

Includes an appendix describing test equipment useful for analog and mixed-signal work.

Examines the basics of linear systems, types of nonlinearities and their effects, op-amp circuits, the high-gain analog filter-amplifier, and signal generation Comprehensive and detailed, Analog and Mixed-Signal Electronics is a great introduction to analog and mixed-signal electronics for EE undergraduates, advanced electronics students, and for those involved in computer engineering, biomedical engineering, computer science, and physics.

Ethical and Otherwise:
Engineering In the Headlines

Karl Stephan

ASIN: B018KQ1K7C
Publication Date: December 7, 2015
Available on Kindle, $6.99
Sold by: Amazon Digital Services LLC
186 pages
Language: English

When engineering or technology shows up in headlines, it's usually because something goes wrong. Since 2006, Karl Stephan has been writing a weekly blog on newsworthy topics in engineering and technology with an ethical angle. This book collects over 40 of his most popular blogs, and covers disasters of many kinds (both modern and historic), blunders and lawbreaking by corporations and individuals, and thoughts on the engineering profession. In the first section, "Tragedies Large and Small," there are chapters describing the sinking of the Titanic, fertilizer explosions at Texas City (1947) and West (2013), as well as air crashes, railroad wrecks, and building and construction failures. In part 2, "Cautionary Tales" the ethics of technological businesses comes under examination. Part 3, "The Engineering Profession," includes matters such as professional licensing, engineering education, and patents.

Each chapter is self-contained with up-to-date references. This book is an excellent reference source for engineering and professional ethics cases, as well as an entertaining read.

Of This Sad Time
My Wife's Journey Through Breast Cancer

Now On Kindle

Karl Stephan

ASIN: B0182Q8U0U
Publication Date: November 25, 2015
Available on Kindle, $3.49
Sold by: Amazon Digital Services LLC
117 pages
Language: English

A diagnosis of breast cancer can be devastating not only for the woman who has it, but for her partner as well. This is a memoir by the husband of a breast-cancer victim who nearly died, not from the disease, but from side effects of the treatment. Faith, help and encouragement from friends, and a new oncologist pulled her through. If you're a man whose wife or girlfriend is facing breast cancer, this book will show you how a self-confessed nerd who couldn't stand the sight of blood discovered resources of courage, persistence, and love that he didn't know he had. Surviving cancer is no picnic, and this book doesn't sugar-coat the risks, dangers, and temptations involved. Whether she admits it or not, a woman with breast cancer needs lots of support, and this story describes how the victim's husband supported her throughout her ordeal, helping her navigate the complexities of diagnosis and treatment options, holding her head while she lost her cookies, and taking up the slack of household chores. Written with clarity, directness, and occasionally humor, this story will inspire couples facing breast cancer with hope, encouragement, and a new sense of purpose.